Understanding Baffling Psychotherapy Clients

Case Studies, Clinical Wisdom, and Lessons from Fifty Years of Practice

Jeff Duffey, MD

Understanding Baffling Psychotherapy Clients: Case Studies, Clinical Wisdom, and Lessons from Fifty Years of Practice

by Jeff Duffey, MD

ISBN 9798993080710 (paperback)

ISBN 9798993080727 (ebook)

ISBN 9798993080734 (audio)

Library of Congress Control Number: 2025919111

First Edition 2026

Edited by Kristy Phillips

Cover by 99 Designs

URLs are provided for informational purposes only, and their mention should not be considered a recommendation. The author is not responsible for the content of these sites. See the disclaimer for more details.

This book is dedicated to all who have taken up the mantle of clinical responsibility.

Contents

Introduction

This book covers the steps to understanding and treating the baffling clients every therapist sees from time to time. It offers anecdotes, vivid illustrations, and insights from my fifty years as a psychiatrist doing psychotherapy.

My training at the Sheppard Pratt Hospital in Baltimore provided me with rare opportunities to learn therapy from experts. I want you to have the advantage of my hard-earned experience and the wisdom they passed along to me.

The initial chapters detail how to find the pieces of history that make up the client puzzle. Subsequent chapters discuss the remaining steps of identifying the client's resistance, uncovering the interplay of feelings between you and the client, discovering the client's dynamics, and employing therapeutic techniques that fit the clinical situation.

In these chapters, the therapeutic relationship will emerge as an essential tool in understanding and treating the client. You will also find more detailed discussions of clients who dissociate, have autism, or endure profound suffering.

By reading *Understanding Baffling Psychotherapy Clients*, you can:

- Benefit from practical tips learned from my fifty-plus years of practicing psychiatry
- Find hidden clues that your baffling client is giving you in their history
- Examine the sources of their resistance to change
- Explore the complexities of your therapeutic relationship
- Discover how your experience in providing therapy compares with others
- Add to your therapy techniques
- Look at valuable basic concepts in a new light
- Consider the spiritual challenge that suffering raises for your client and for you as the person who sits with them in their suffering

I wrote this book especially for counselors, marriage and family therapists, social workers, psychologists, psychiatric nurses, psychiatrists, and others who provide therapy. This book's useful medical information helps everyone who provides therapy better understand the whole client.

The first chapters are packed with instructive pointers, similar to textbooks or educational materials that you are familiar with. If you need to pause from taking in all the information, consider skipping ahead to later chapters that spark your interest. Then return to the first chapters later.

None of us is perfect, and it takes time and experience to fully embrace the idea that therapy does not have to be perfect to work. In the stories I share, you will read about some of the mistakes I have made. Perhaps they will help you relax and not worry so much about your own imperfection. Remember: Witnessing your self-acceptance will help your clients accept themselves.

I hope this book will continue to resonate even more with you when you reference it after collecting more experiences.

When you study *Understanding Your Baffling Psychotherapy Clients*, I believe you will further develop the three C's that are the hallmarks of sound therapy: caring, competence, and carefulness. Increasing those in your practice will bring you more of another C: confidence.

Additional resources and links to citations and references can be found on my website: jeffduffeymdbooks.com

Disclaimer

Life and people are messy. They have a lovely sloppiness that spills over precise categories and defies absolutes. Difficult to pin down, they frustrate our wish for simple answers and reward us with fascinating complexity. It's no wonder many of the statements you will read in this book have qualifiers. Life varies. People vary. So brace yourself for the frequent use of *sometimes, some, may, occasionally, often, at times*, and *might*. Although they may make some sentences cumbersome, these words reflect the varied nature of what I describe.

My offering you advice implies that I know what is best for you in the same way your advice implies that you know what is best for your client. I cannot presume that I know what is best for you or your unique situations. These tips are additional options for you to consider, not directives.

As I wrote this book, I imagined myself talking openly to you about what I find central in providing therapy. Sometimes, you may hear me raise my voice. Those will be times when I am worried for you because I know how dire the consequences of a particular mistake might be.

For the sake of simplicity, I use *him*, *her*, or *they* when it seems applicable.

Also, this book embraces more than the medical model of treatment. So I use *client* instead of *patient* when discussing people in treatment unless those people are in the hospital.

You will see my point of view shift when I refer in general to therapy, medical information, or legal matters.

Please apply to this book the same critical-thinking skills you use when you read journals and research articles.

Even though I hope you do not have any problems as a result of reading this book, I take no responsibility for how this book affects you. I also take no responsibility for any decisions you make after reading it.

Although the publisher and I have made every effort to ensure accuracy and completeness, we cannot guarantee or warrant that the contents of this book are accurate, up-to-date, or complete. We also cannot be responsible for any third-party resources discussed in this book.

The information provided is intended to help you make better, more informed decisions in your practice. It is not a substitute for formal professional education, medical advice, or treatment. I cannot give you medical advice, and I urge you to consult your physician before making any decisions regarding health-related matters.

Similarly, the information in this book is not a substitute for legal advice from a licensed attorney, and you should not consider anything in this book a solicitation of legal advice. If you have any legal questions or concerns, you should consult an attorney licensed in your state.

To preserve my clients' confidentiality, I have significantly changed or omitted identifiable client information. Many of the client cases are constructed from composites of multiple clients. Any resemblance to people, living or dead, is purely coincidental.

Part 1

GATHERING NEEDED INFORMATION

This section is devoted to the various elements that go into history taking and the clues that you can discover from taking a thorough history.

Chapter 1

Unearthing Clients' Strengths

When you ask questions to help your client solve their personal puzzle, it is not just what you ask, but how you ask that matters. Focusing on your client's strengths and examples of their agency empowers them with hope, even as you discover their problems.

Therapy is an enthralling experience.

As a therapist, you share in one of the few situations in life in which people talk frankly about intensely personal feelings and experiences. What an adventure psychotherapy is. You get the opportunity to know someone well, watch them grow and heal, and discover the difference you can make in their life. No two workdays are alike. Your work explodes with discoveries and techniques, making the work intellectually satisfying. Being a therapist is exciting.

Clients are excited, too, at the prospect of feeling better. On their way to a session, clients sometimes talk to the therapist in their mind. They rehearse what they want to say. In the session, they may have a kind of selective attention. The concerns that occupy their mind and stir their emotions can narrow their perceptions of the surroundings. They may be too distracted to remember important information.

My wife taught me that I could save time in the morning by pouring Cheerios into a cup and covering them with milk. I learned to drink breakfast in the car at stoplights on my way to work. All along, the Cheerios got stickier and stickier. So I would shake my cup harder and harder, tossing the loosened Cheerios into my mouth.

One day, I took a bathroom break after seeing clients all morning. Looking into the mirror, I saw a Cheerio lodged squarely in the nosepiece of my glasses. No one had said a thing. I suspect they were so focused on their concerns that they looked right at me and didn't see it. Perhaps clients who did were too polite to tell me how silly I looked. I will never know.

The therapeutic setting's intensity affects your focus as well. Your experience and the person you are influence how working with clients affects you. Each therapist's experience is unique, as is each therapeutic situation.

This chapter's many questions about the initial interview are appropriate for the first interview. However, time limitations may force you to postpone some questions to a later session. In the first interview, focus on discovering what you need to know to make that session's decisions and on helping your client feel safe.

At the beginning of the interview, explain the purpose of your initial interview and your goals for this first part of treatment. Knowing what to expect helps your client feel safe. They know what to expect and are less likely to be surprised.

Offset the effect of uncovering the client's weaknesses by discussing their strengths.

For example, point out their strengths by commending them for filling out the forms, putting up with waiting for the appointment, getting up early, dealing with the traffic, or overcoming any other obstacles they faced in seeing you. These comments immediately highlight the strengths they have already shown and their ability to overcome problems.

Perhaps your client reveals that they have suffered the ill effects of being bullied. Ask about how they developed the courage to persist and what they learned about their inner strength. How did they successfully apply what they learned when they faced a similar situation? You do this to highlight the agency they have shown.

Clients may see themselves as having traits similar to their parents'. If you help them identify the qualities they like in their parents, you reinforce the parents' positive aspects that the client has internalized.

Let's say your client's parent persisted in the face of adversity. Discussing this may boost your client's confidence so they will not give up trying.

Find examples of your client's agency.

When a client discusses a crisis, point out that they have already survived their earlier hard times and learned from them, so it is reasonable to believe they will master the current situation. Be sure to find parts of their life that are going well and are not affected by their presenting problem. Ask about times when they were discouraged but experienced a change that improved things over time.

As they share their school and job histories, highlight their accomplishments and the lessons they have learned. Identify ways they became better with practice and effort. Reframe their mistakes as part of the normal process of learning by trial and error. Stress that they are not fixed entities and can grow and change like everyone can.

Reframe to help them develop an interesting vision of how outcomes might be different.

When you spark their positive thinking, you counterbalance your questions about shortcomings.

For example, a client may beat themselves up over a romantic relationship that did not work out. Did they show social skills and maturity in coping with a difficult partner? Did they help the partner grow despite the relationship ending? Could breaking up represent a growing belief in their self-worth? Help them look for the silver lining in the storm clouds.

When appropriate, normalize their experience without minimizing their distress. For example, if they are having trouble sleeping, empathize with how annoying it is to lack sleep, even though it is not uncommon. Ask if they have tried something that helped. Get them to imagine what it would be like if they didn't have the difficulty.

When describing the presenting problem and treatment plan, use words that reflect optimism and a positive mindset.

Collaborate with your client to develop a treatment plan without guaranteeing specific results. This future-oriented perspective shows that you believe they can recover by taking these positive steps.

Some of the client's presenting issues result from a brain/body illness with a specific diagnosis and treatment. So you can't overlook a medical aspect of mental illness in your evaluation. And you still must ask about physical symptoms.

Having a symptom implies the client is the passive object of something going wrong. Even when that is only somewhat true, you want to stress that your client is a partner in treating their illness. You want to continue to nourish their agency and positive aspirations. Hope promotes cooperation, making it more likely that your client will continue treatment.

Let's say you investigate a client's sleep problems and uncover the classic signs and symptoms of sleep apnea. The sleep workup confirms the diagnosis. Your client may feel relieved to have a diagnosis with specific, successful treatments. The diagnosis does not threaten their self-view or stigmatize them.

A different client may be physically well but have mental problems behind their sleep issues. If you list the goal as treating insomnia, it implies a concrete, static condition. Instead, frame the goal in more fluid terms. Describe the goals as developing better sleep patterns, maximizing conditions that promote sleep, and dealing with stressors. In this way, you show your client that you believe they have a path to recovery rather than a static condition to suffer with.

As you approach the initial interview, take comfort in common things happening most commonly. Your experience and training will help you identify those common patterns and successfully treat them. The occasional client who surprises you by being so different from what you expected will keep you on your toes. As you know, clients often have a mixture of both physical and mental issues. One may magnify the effects of the other. With practice, you will become more comfortable interviewing clients with both.

In this chapter: We discussed the importance of framing questions, client issues, and future treatment in positive terms to foster a positive mindset in your client.

In the next chapter: We'll examine your preparations before you sit down with your client. You will consider how different techniques produce different outcomes, how visual clues and outside information make for a more reliable assessment, and the importance of knowing about ancestral stress. In Chapter 2, you will read for the first time about PODS and how you can use it to remember to ask the most clinically relevant questions as you work to understand your baffling client.

Chapter 2
Collecting Information Before Your Initial Evaluation

Your client's history has many implications. How you structure the interview makes a difference. Frame your questions to underscore strengths. Double-check the accuracy of what you are told. Inspect your client and how they answered the questionnaire.

You may want to read an even more comprehensive, detailed discussion of the diagnostic interview: *The Psychiatric Interview in Clinical Practice* by Roger A. MacKinnon, MD; Robert Michels, MD; and Peter J. Buckley, MD (American Psychiatric Publishing, Washington, DC, and London, England).

Different interview techniques optimize different outcomes.

If you do an interview to try to understand the client's psychodynamics, it will be significantly less structured. In that way, you lessen your influence on the client's process and can see more clearly what is happening. Suppose you are trying to decide on medical treatment by identifying symptoms and making a diagnosis that will lead to a specific treatment course. In that case, your interview will follow a more structured medical model. That model is more consistent with doing supportive psychotherapy together with psychopharmacology.

Say a physician has thoroughly examined a client and declared them to be physically healthy. Assume also that they can afford to see you for a significant amount of time and will commit to therapy for as long as they need it and as often as required. They don't have a substance abuse problem and are convincingly not suicidal. If all these criteria are met, you have the basis for insight-oriented psychotherapy that is much less structured and better reflects the patient.

Have you ever watched a murder mystery where a bystander carelessly contaminates the crime scene before the forensic team can examine it to figure out what happened? You might feel like that bystander when you use a more directive approach to interviewing. Everything said can feel like another fingerprint that might obscure an underlying process.

More directive interviewing is a compromise when you need to be practical in a less-than-ideal situation. A more direct approach is done at the expense of something else. Instead of the client telling you what they want from their history, you ask for details about their history, possibly leaving out something more important to them. It better reflects *your* ideas and judgments about what is essential. It may lead to a mistaken conclusion that would have been different with more information.

When you take a less direct approach, you may fail to identify potential health issues and essential medical history. Then you may be in the dark about something serious and perhaps even dangerous.

As I now discuss the mechanics of what I learned about the more directive method of taking a history, remember that the technique has limits:

- Is your client's history accurate?
- Is their story plausible?
- Does it fit with the information you have from other sources?
- Are they hiding information because they are worried you might commit them to a hospital involuntarily?
- Is a psychotic process interfering with their perception of reality? Are they exaggerating symptoms to get disability benefits?
- Is there a history of others not believing they are suffering, so they must endorse every symptom as a cry for help?

A client may say something that sounds ridiculous. Check it out anyway. For example, I saw a forensic inpatient who told me he was feeling good because he had just come from singing Christmas carols. It was July. I found that a volunteer group had been at the hospital and put on their Christmas program during the only time they had available.

I have worked with clients who had dissociative identity disorder (formerly referred to as multiple personality disorder). They were not aware of their actions or inactions when another alter (alternative personality) was in consciousness.

One client told me they were about to take a drug test for work when another alter told them they couldn't do that because they used marijuana. This was a surprise to the prim and proper alter who was a professional.

Getting an accurate sexual and contraceptive history can be a problem when working with dissociative clients with alters who have unprotected intercourse. Not only do they risk pregnancy and sexually transmitted diseases, but they may also take medications that cause fetal harm, and you don't know whether they are forgetting to use birth control.

Client interviews are often conducted under challenging conditions. There may be inadequate privacy, uncomfortable surroundings, and unreasonable limits on session length. Therapy might have to be done in cramped, noisy, hastily provided spaces in schools, homes, or public buildings. (Be careful that you are not isolated. Ensure that there are people around who could later confirm that your behavior was always appropriate.)

Poorly designed electronic medical records may compound the difficulty by requiring you to check boxes and limiting free text space. Paradigms that don't fit may point you in the wrong direction and make it harder to think more broadly.

These conditions can make it challenging to do your best and may make you feel compromised. Under these conditions, it would be helpful to differentiate what you can control. Don't let perfectionism rob you of feeling satisfied that you did what you could with what was available. Show yourself some mercy and grace.

Please think of the client as a flower that opens its petals with the sunlight and closes quickly without it. Active listening is the sunlight. The client may need extra time to say what they feel compelled to say. That may cut into the time you need to find out what else you should know. Within reason, the client's wishes should come first.

The first thing the patient talks about is likely what they care about most. Listen carefully and give them an empathic gift by clearly state what they just said. When time requires a more direct approach, apologize before beginning your questions.

Fortunately, with practice, you can learn which questions are clinically most relevant to ask in your limited time. I like to use the acronym PODS, which stands for **p**sychotic, **o**rganic, **d**rug-affected/**d**epressed, and **s**uicidal. (Many conditions can cause a psychotic state. Very simply, a client in a psychotic state is disconnected from reality and may hold incorrect beliefs, called delusions. They may have hallucinations, in which they hear or see things that are not there.)

When I am pressed for time, my interview questions are directed first at identifying whether the client is psychotic, organic, drug-affected/depressed, or suicidal. I remind myself to expect the unexpected, so I don't overlook it. More about the elements that make up PODS is scattered throughout the book.

Corroborate sources of information.

Before meeting your client, read any available client record. Ask your client to sign a release to get information from past treaters. This practice is the standard of care. Knowing what has worked before can also help you make decisions. Other sources may reveal long-standing patterns of client behavior. There could be things in the record that the client did not have time to mention, may have forgotten, or wanted to hide. If your client refuses to sign a release, document that you made the request and they declined.

When a family member, partner, or friend accompanies the client, take advantage of what they know. It is particularly important to ask them about any history of the client having symptoms of mania or hypomania. Bipolar I and II disorders are often misdiagnosed as depression because the client presents when they are depressed and does not experience the manic symptoms as a problem.

Family members may not know what a manic episode or a particular diagnostic picture looks like. You might first ask about specific symptoms they may have noticed, like excessive energy and less need for sleep. Perhaps they remember the client taking lithium or having a side effect that suggests the client was on antipsychotic medication.

During a more medically oriented interview, ask both individuals to come in before the client can confide anything to you. Explain that you will see the client but that you first want to hear the family member's concerns. Explain that you cannot tell the family member anything without the client's permission, but they are free to tell you what they wish.

With your client still present, some of your questions may need to be delicate and indirect. For example, rather than asking the family member if the client abuses drugs, ask about withdrawal symptoms or times when the client kept to themselves, missed activities, had sudden bursts of appetite, or seemed unusually forgetful or unmotivated. Ask about changes in behavior and indirect indications that might suggest suicidal risk.

Watch the interaction between the client and the family member. Thank the family member and allow them to leave the office alone so the client is assured that you have spent no time alone with the other person, talking behind the client's back.

Explain to your client that therapy is a collaborative enterprise, but you must be more direct during the initial interview.

When you don't have the luxury of having family or friends present, ask the client how people close to them perceive their presenting concerns.

Consider what your patient tells you as basically accurate until proven otherwise.

A client may reveal history that seems self-serving, exaggerated, far-fetched, or so different from your own experience that you have trouble believing it. I did not have an open mind when I listened to my client Althea, and there were consequences.

Althea did not have time to wear makeup or do her hair before our sessions. She had two young children to care for, cooking to do, and a house to keep clean. In sessions, she continually complained about how inadequate her husband was. He was not much of a provider, and Althea asked if they could barter work in exchange for my services. Despite not wanting that to be an artifact in therapy, I compromised by having Althea's husband, not her, do the work. He was to report to my wife and not deal with me. Althea agreed, and he came to our farm.

Within days, our chickens stopped laying eggs. We could not figure it out. My wife had given Althea's husband clear and detailed instructions. He had not followed them properly and had put up black plastic, not transparent plastic, over all the chicken coop windows. It was now always night for the chickens. There was no shift from nighttime to daytime for the chicken's brains to know it was time to lay eggs. I should have listened more closely to Althea's complaints and believed her.

It isn't just what the client says that is relevant. It is also everything you see.

There may be a quote on a T-shirt, a commemorative phrase tattooed on an arm, visible relief when a family member leaves, or a wedding ring still on a widower's finger.

Observing how your client walks down the hall to your office may be a clue about their arthritis, orthopedic problem, old injury, chronic back pain, or excessive mobility of their joints. Look for signs of asymmetry, which may suggest ill health. For example, do they favor one side? Do they bite their fingernails? Are their fingers nicotine-stained?

Therapists skilled in neurolinguistic programming have added skills in watching a client's eye movements to gain insight into what kind of information they are accessing in their brain (Bandler and Grinder 1979).

Here are examples of signs to consider:

- Perhaps you see dilated pupils in people using cannabis and psychostimulants, including methamphetamine (sometimes referred to as "meth"). People using opiates and barbiturates may have constricted pupils. Could the client be high in the interview? Did they worry they would not relax enough without using substances?
- Ask about a visible tremor. It could be a benign familial tremor that runs in families. It may be a sign of anxiety, the effect of medication, the impact of withdrawing from medication/alcohol, or stemming from several other causes, including serious neurological diseases.
- If the client is noticeably overweight, consider whether they could have silent inflammation, an immunological reaction characterized by a less obvious chronic inflammatory process that occurs at a cellular level. Silent inflammation is not uncommon and is behind multiple diseases. It can contribute to depression. David Furman et al.'s article, "Chronic inflammation in the etiology of disease across the life span," explains how chronic inflammation affects the body (Furman et al. 2019).
- If your client dresses in baggy clothes, could they have an eating disorder and be hiding a skinny body?
- If they dress in clothes that minimize their sexuality, could they have been the victim of sexual abuse? Some abused clients who felt vulnerable because of their small size later bulk up to feel bigger and safer.
- If they dress seductively, do they see their worth or power coming from their appearance?

- If they have body odor, are they so depressed that they are not doing activities of daily living? Could their offensive odor be a subtle way of showing contempt?
- Does their breath smell like alcohol? Is there a hint of the smell of acetone, which smells like nail polish and suggests ketosis from diabetes or a keto diet? (Ketones result from the breakdown of fat when glucose is not readily available. Ketosis is the presence of many ketones in the blood.)

Remotely interviewing clients has its own set of considerations. Typically, you can see clients with the hyperactivity of attention deficit hyperactivity disorder (ADHD) moving during the interview. If you see them remotely, ask if they are moving their body outside of view.

Client movement is not the only situation you might miss when you see someone remotely. One young woman I saw remotely said she was alone at home. However, as the interview progressed, it seemed she was becoming more guarded. It became clear later when her mother, who had entered her room, asked a question.

Another young woman did not show up for her remote 9:30 a.m. appointment. When I called her, she said she would get online. A few minutes later, she came on the screen wearing pajamas and sitting on her bed. She told me she was having trouble getting restful sleep. I thought about sleep apnea, a condition in which breathing intermittently stops during sleep. When I asked whether anyone had seen her stop breathing while she was asleep, a voice came from the other side of the bed. Her boyfriend said, "She doesn't quit breathing in her sleep."

When you have an urgent situation and can't examine the client in person, consider enlisting a family member's help. They may see a tremor you can't, smell alcohol on the client's breath, look for dilated pupils, describe a rash in more detail, and, with enough instruction, check for cogwheeling rigidity in a client on antipsychotic medication. The information may not be as accurate, but it is worth getting.

You may notice that you have access to other ways to observe a client. I once interviewed a man in the intensive care unit (ICU). I could see his electrocardiogram (EKG) monitor in the background. When I asked him about his sister, he started throwing irregular heartbeats. I changed the subject, and his heartbeat became regular again.

Ask about ancestral stress and maternal postpartum depression.

Be mindful that factors affecting your client may have started before or around their birth. Preliminary research suggests that trauma to a client's ancestors can cause epigenetic changes—environmentally or behaviorally induced changes in how genes work. Yehuda and Lehrner spell it out in their article "Intergenerational transmission of trauma effects: Putative role of epigenetic mechanisms" (Yehuda and Lehrner 2018).

What does the client know about their mother's pregnancy and the conditions surrounding their birth? The client may have been exposed while in the uterus to their mother's stress.

Perhaps family members have told your client that their mother had postpartum depression and could not bond with your client.

There are clues in how the client completes the questionnaire.

If the client completes a questionnaire before the interview, it will unintentionally shape the interview narrative by revealing what you value. It's like throwing a pebble into still water.

I have used a comprehensive questionnaire and accepted the trade-off because of my work parameters. The questionnaire matches the sections of my report. I ask for it to be returned early so I can study it before the interview. Because it is extensive, it saves time and reduces the chances of overlooking an important detail during a time-limited session.

A questionnaire interferes with your chance to see a client's thought process. However, completing the questionnaire requires them to explain what is happening. Their description of the problem reflects what is consciously available to them.

How they answer a form also gives you a glimpse of their cognitive abilities and, perhaps, general knowledge. You may notice limited vocabulary, poor spelling, grammatical errors, poorly organized responses, or sloppy handwriting. Their written responses could reflect an inability to understand the questions or grasp what is being asked. These are all clues about their ability to solve problems and their level of motivation. Could their difficulties in functioning suggest they had limited educational opportunities, have a learning disorder or attentional problems, or are on the autistic spectrum?

If they give cursory or inconsistent responses, it may mean they lack commitment, are hiding something, or have a flippant attitude.

If they show up without completing the form, there could be multiple reasons. Maybe they were pressured to see you. It may be a sign they are passive-aggressive or oppositional. Perhaps they expect an exception to be made. Or their life is unmanageable.

Excessively detailed responses might suggest a tendency to obsess, perfectionism, or the need to avoid expected criticism by doing it just right. They may also not want to be misunderstood or have you miss a detail.

In this chapter: I showed how multiple sources can supplement what your client tells you. Topics included the effect of different interviewing techniques on the information you get and the importance of visual clues, including how the client dresses and moves. I mentioned the role of ancestral stressors and postpartum depression. All may contribute to your client's baffling condition.

In the next chapter: We'll shift the time frame to the present and more recent past. Major puzzle pieces come from your client's description of what bothers them most. In obtaining the treatment history, you see where the mines are in the therapy minefield because the last therapist stepped on some.

Chapter 3

Getting a History of Present and Past Psychiatric Illness

Please focus on the client's view of why they are coming for treatment. Their response to past treatment, medication, and surgery may predict their response to future treatment. Their psychiatric medication history may guide treatment decisions.

Present illness and chief complaint reflect what concerns your client most.

I find it exciting to take a client's history. I am a detective looking for clues about what is going on. Clients are unaware of their own unconscious resistance, so they welcome your collaboration in solving their problem. Thankful for the opportunity to express their feelings, they relish having someone attentively listen. They may take comfort in feeling no longer alone in their struggle.

It is essential to understand when the client's suffering began. Your client's suffering is new to you, and you are naturally hopeful. But your client may be worn out, having already tried many things without success. Without a clear idea of the onset, you don't know how much time you have left in the game before the client becomes unwilling to continue therapy or their life. The time left could be dangerously short.

In taking a present illness, listen for evidence of recent trauma. Examples of trauma include sexual assault, physical assault, natural disasters, abuse, traumatic accidents, and combat.

Or the trauma may be an ongoing situation in which the client is deprived of something positive. They may lack food, warmth, shelter, love, parenting, or freedom.

When your client cannot identify an obvious cause of their current suffering, look for a trigger that caused them to reexperience a past suffering or trauma. For example, a mother who was raped on her prom night might be triggered by her daughter's upcoming prom.

When you ask what prompted them to see you, notice their word choices and tone of voice:

- Do they use passive voice as though they had no agency?
- As they talk about their current situation, listen for clues to who loved them and whom they loved.
- What they emphasize could be a sign of what they value. Do they focus on their losses, failures, and regrets? This might be expected in a client with a negative mindset.
- Do the symptoms seem to come in cycles? How long do the cycles last?

- Must there be a situational trigger?
- How disabling are the symptoms?

Distinguishing affective instability (unstable moods), bipolar disorder type II, bipolar disorder type I, mixed states, and drug/medication-induced mood changes is tricky because symptoms overlap. Michael G. Pipich, MS, LMFT, helps clarify this in his *Psychology Today* article: "Bipolar and Borderline: A Differential Roadmap" (Pipich 2020).

Bipolar clients most often present with depression, and it is easy to misdiagnose them. It is generally accepted that treating a bipolar client with an antidepressant is ineffective and may make them worse. This makes it even more important to look for evidence of a history of mania, hypomania, or mixed features.

When your client complains of anxiety and depression symptoms, ask them first about times when they felt unusually talkative, energetic, and positive, as though things could not be better. In this way, you may find out about past periods of hypomania or mania. They may have had mixed features, which is having symptoms of both mania and depression at the same time.

Past psychiatric treatment in both inpatient and outpatient settings predicts future problems.

The quality of inpatient psychiatric treatment facilities differs. Inpatient treatment can be disturbingly traumatic or life-saving and wonderful. Ask:

- About how long did the provider typically spend with the client?
- Did the provider have time to get to know them?
- Did the client respond to the treatments?
- What medications were prescribed and successfully swallowed?
- What did the client learn from the experience?
- Was the family included in the treatment?
- Was the client overmedicated?
- Did they have side effects because the dose was raised too quickly?
- Were medications given a long enough time frame to work before being changed?
- What was the hospital milieu like?

Ask similar questions about outpatient treatment. Be especially concerned with whether the psychiatric treaters were thorough and thoughtful in their approach or whether treatment was haphazard and based on brief, perfunctory visits. Therapists are usually given more time to spend with clients than doctors, see them more often, and have a better chance of getting to know them well.

Take an interest in any history of a lack of cooperation. For example, your client might miss medications or appointments. They may have failed to do homework assignments a previous provider gave as part of treatment. Those indicators give you an idea of what to expect from the client in the future.

If the client formed a positive working alliance with the therapist, had a good outcome, and dealt with the termination (the ending of therapy) well, they are more likely to succeed in future therapies. If it was unsuccessful, you might want to spend extra effort building a better treatment alliance than they had with the past therapist. This additional effort might mean taking more time up-front to spell out expectations and educate the patient about treatment, procedures, and rationale.

Past psychiatric medication history maps some of the medical minefield.

The medications your client is taking or has taken may explain their current situation. For example, certain antidepressants and some other drugs may cause affective blunting, which is a reduced emotional reactivity and a sense of numbness. At first glance, that can look like anhedonia, where the client can't enjoy enjoyable things.

Affective blunting may also be part of a more complicated amotivational syndrome. Both antidepressants and marijuana can cause an amotivational syndrome that will impair the client's progress. A client with this syndrome may seem generally disinterested, unemotional, removed from what is happening, and forgetful.

Is it possible that the prescriber used too high a dose of the antidepressant? You may want to discuss whether the prescriber needs to use a medication with a different mechanism of action. Sometimes, prescribers add a differently acting medication for balance.

When a client does not improve or gets worse after an adequate antidepressant trial, reconsider whether a bipolar illness has been overlooked. Clients may fail to recall a period of several days of hypomanic behavior that they experienced as being more productive. Asking the family about such episodes could prove pivotal for future treatment.

Your client's past response to medication provides direction for future treatment. For example, improvement on one medication and not another can give you an idea about how they metabolize (digest) medications. There are different metabolic pathways. Clients may have inherited the ability to go quickly on one pathway and slowly on another. Medication may be metabolized on one or multiple pathways.

If your client has a history of not responding to a medication, they may be a fast metabolizer on the pathway used to metabolize that drug. They get the drug out of their body fast. So they need a higher dose to keep the drug's level in their blood at a therapeutic level.

If your client has excessive side effects from a particular drug, they may be a slow metabolizer of that medication and have too much medication in their blood.

You could ask your clinician to order a genetic test battery related to psychotropic medications (medications that affect the brain) to see how your client's genetics affect how they metabolize specific drugs. GeneSight is one of several companies that do genetic testing. Visit its website to learn more. https://genesight.com/for-clinicians/

Genetic testing helps take some of the trial and error out of prescribing. It can alert you to problems with the serotonin transport system associated with higher suicide risk. (Serotonin is a neurotransmitter or messenger chemical in the brain.)

Finally, if your client had an allergic reaction to a particular class of medication, avoid other medications in that class. For example, an allergy to a cephalosporin antibiotic might suggest the client would be allergic to another antibiotic in the cephalosporin class.

In this chapter: I addressed some hidden elements. Could they explain your baffling client? Perhaps different metabolism, inept past treatment, genetic differences, or nonadherence are part of the picture.

In the next chapter: We'll talk about the risk of suicide and violence. I'll provide a list of items that need to be removed from potentially suicidal clients and a brief discussion of unbearable feeling states that risk suicide. I also recommend some excellent articles, some of which will help you assess both general suicide risk and post-discharge risk. Others will address unbearable feeling states and determine the risk of violence.

Chapter 4

Taking a History
of Suicide Risk

*Understanding the risks of future suicidal behavior and
the most alarming symptoms is essential.*

**The risk of suicide spikes in the weeks just
after discharge from inpatient treatment.**

Because of the increased risk, it is essential to know how long
ago the inpatient treatment took place. Learn in some detail
what led to the client's hospitalization. Lana Bojanic et al.
discussed this in "Early Post-Discharge Suicide in Mental
Health Patients: Findings from a National Clinical Survey"
(Bojanic et al. 2020).

Be sure to ask whether firearms are unloaded and securely
locked. If you feel there is a risk of suicide, ask if you can talk
to a family member or friend. Ask them to help your client
remove or securely hold those firearms and other possible
dangerous items. Dangerous items might include:

- Prescription and over-the-counter medications
- Poisons
- Antifreeze
- Household cleaners
- Matches
- Inhalants
- Electric cords
- Ropes
- Belts
- Plastic bags
- Sharp items (knives, razors, and kitchen utensils)
- Vehicles (which could be used to crash or to cause carbon monoxide poisoning)

Double-check that the helper followed your recommendations. Emphasize to the helper that they must contact you before releasing the firearms or other items. Make sure the support system has your contact information.

Helping your client overcome their sense of shame at having suicidal thoughts is a first step to helping them open up. Talk about how ordinary people may have suicidal thoughts in different situations and give some examples.

Ask them about their experience and how they manage their thoughts. This opens a conversation and signals that you're comfortable talking. It implies that you don't see the client as the inevitable victim of suicidal thinking. If they have had previous attempts, ask them what they have learned that might help them handle thoughts in the future. This question suggests that something positive can come out of past attempts.

Some clients might find it even harder to talk about their suicidal thoughts with family members than with you. You might ask your client about times when they were surprised by someone's acceptance and forgiveness. For example, did your client ever wreck a car, fail a class, get into a fight, do something embarrassing in public, or break the law but found that their parents pushed past their disappointment to understand them?

Rather than debating with your client the futility of talking to family, focus on the how and emphasize that you will be with your client to help present their side. Ask them what it would be like to learn that they had underestimated a loved one's ability to understand and accept them. Encourage them to imagine what it would be like to realize they no longer need to feel alienated.

The symptoms of frantic hopelessness, ruminative flooding, and near-psychotic somatization require you to take immediate action.

Some symptoms require you to take immediate action when you hear about them because they could be short-term predictors of suicide.

The following is from an article titled "Is It Possible to Assess Short-Term Risk of Suicide?":

> Dr. Igor Galynker developed a tool to identify when a person is in what he calls a "suicide trigger state." According to Dr. Galynker, the main elements of the

"suicide trigger state" (STS) include "ruminative flooding" and "frantic hopelessness." Ruminative flooding refers to when a person has rapid and repeated negative thoughts that are both confusing and difficult to stop. Frantic hopelessness refers to the feeling that life will always be painful and unchangeable, along with an overwhelming feeling of being "trapped." This combination of thoughts and feelings can trigger suicidal behavior (American Foundation for Suicide Prevention 2018).

Later, a third item was added, which is "near-psychotic somatic delusions." *(Somatic* refers to the body. A somatic delusion is a false belief about the body. Somatization is a defense against anxiety that directs mental distress into physical symptoms. Instead of experiencing the anxiety, the client experiences it as a physical symptom.)

In a *Psychiatric Times* article called "Can a Suicide Scale Predict the Unpredictable?" Arline Kaplan wrote:

> All of this builds, they added, to an intolerable, confused state in which patients feel that suicidal action is the only conceivable route of escape. In this state of severe distress, many patients have also reported the experience of 'near-psychotic somatization,' characterized by feeling as if their thoughts are creating head pressure (e.g., feeling as if the head was going to explode), as well as some somatic distortions (e.g., change in body size or shape) (Kaplan 2011).

Researchers have used the Suicide Trigger Scale in the emergency room. This scale is discussed in an article titled "Emergency room validation of the revised Suicide Trigger Scale (STS-3): a measure of a hypothesized suicide trigger state" (Yaseen et al. 2012).

A significant percentage of clients with narcolepsy have considered suicide. Their depressive symptoms, inattentiveness, avoidance of strong emotion that could trigger catalepsy, and difficulty sleeping at night may overshadow their excessive daytime sleepiness and look more like some combination of depression, ADHD, and social anxiety.

Being unable to resist sleep in the daytime—which is the more characteristic symptom of narcolepsy—and the episodic loss of autonomic muscle tone characteristic of catalepsy can be hidden by symptoms resembling more frequent diagnoses.

Self-injury is not synonymous with suicidal behavior. You can find a comprehensive discussion of non-suicidal self-injurious behavior in the article titled "Nonsuicidal Self-Injury: Diagnostic Challenges And Current Perspectives" (Hooley et al. 2020). https://pmc.ncbi.nlm.nih.gov/articles/PMC6959491/

Assessing violence risk is critical but beyond the scope of this book.

It bears repeating that while treatment encourages clients to recognize their agency, your client may have lived in a situation that realistically limited their freedom of choice. They may not have been able to act the way they would like to for fear of endangering their family's safety or health, going hungry, or losing their way to make a living.

They may have regrets about things they have had to do to survive. Considering their political, social, and financial situations will help you talk with them about the myriad feelings involved in choosing between the lesser of two bad choices. Again, when you listen sympathetically to how they feel about their compromising situations, you show the mercy you would like them to show themselves and reduce their unrealistic shame. Shame can feel unbearable and contribute to suicidal risk.

In this chapter: The key takeaway is to understand that frantic hopelessness, ruminative flooding, and near-psychotic somatization need to be addressed immediately.

In the next chapter: Perhaps the reason you can't make sense of your baffling client's presentation is that they are showing early signs of delirium or a psychotic process. Next, I'll cover the biological and situational factors behind psychosis and delirium.

Chapter 5

Considering Connections That Can Lead to Psychosis

Both organic and situational factors can contribute to the client becoming psychotic.

Identify medical causes and other possible risk factors for psychosis and altered mental status.

Ask about medical illnesses or situations that are associated with psychosis. The Cleveland Clinic addresses these in its article titled "Psychosis." https://my.clevelandclinic.org/health/symptoms/23012-psychosis

Instead of discussing the psychosis-associated illnesses and situations you need to ask about in the history, I want to give examples of how interconnected biological and situational factors are when it comes to altering mental status.

Sometimes, a past surgery or medical event sets the client up for a later neuropsychiatric condition. I did a hospital consultation on a middle-aged business professional who was hospitalized after becoming psychotic. Because of her business acumen, the business community sought her out for advice. This change in her mental status surprised those around her.

She gave a history of having gastric surgery that resulted in the loss of part of her stomach. The stomach absorbs vitamin B12. With less stomach, she could absorb less vitamin B12. So, she was eating things rich in vitamin B12 but not absorbing enough. Vitamin B12 is a necessary coenzyme in creating neurotransmitters. Vitamin B12 deficiency is sometimes associated with psychosis. I was astonished at how quickly her psychosis remitted after her vitamin B12 was restored.

The association between physical deterioration from chronic alcohol addiction, a subsequent fall, and a subdural hematoma is another example of a medical condition possibly causing later neuropsychiatric symptoms. Excessive alcohol use alters balance, which may lead to falls. A fall may cause a subdural hematoma, which is a collection of blood outside the brain. The subdural hematoma can manifest with neuropsychiatric symptoms. When you get a client with a history of excessive drinking, ask about a history of falls and head trauma, which could be behind the symptoms you are seeing.

Falls are not the only source of head trauma. Traumatic brain injury from domestic abuse is also associated with subdural hematomas and neurological symptoms. Your questions about symptoms of traumatic brain injury and multiple concussions should logically follow if your client tells you about domestic abuse.

Infections can also alter mental status. Delirium is a transient alteration in mental status. It can occur in older people who have urinary tract infections. An older adult with new-onset mental changes may warrant urine testing before you seriously consider a psychotic or dementing process.

In this chapter: I shared examples of interconnection that illustrate the need to recognize the interplay of biological and situational factors when a client's history suggests altered mental status, including psychosis and delirium.

In the next chapter: I shift from gathering more psychological information to looking at the part medical illness can play in a client's presentation. I give examples of widely different diseases that might impair a client's mental function.

Chapter 6

Obtaining a Medical History

Physical illness may cause or exacerbate your client's presenting symptoms. Rather than reviewing these illnesses here, I refer you to the questionnaire at the back of this book, which reviews symptoms associated with diseases most likely to cause mental problems.

The new onset of psychiatric symptoms in a client over forty warrants a workup for physical causes. You should suspect physical causes in clients with abnormalities of cognition, speech, and gait, as well as in anyone taking multiple medications. Visual, tactile, and olfactory (smell) hallucinations may have a physical basis.

If your client has not already had a recent physical with appropriate lab work, consider recommending one.

Sometimes, being pushy is necessary and even helpful.

While you may not be the treating physician and not feel like an expert on physical illness, your input into your client's physical treatment may make all the difference. This is particularly true when treating depression, which often has a physical component.

When you are seeing a client with symptoms of depression, it's worth finding out what tests their clinician has already ordered to look for biological causes. You may want to push the clinician to consider testing for thyroid disease, anemia, diabetes, and low testosterone. The clinician may look for sleep apnea, vitamin B12, vitamin D, or other nutritional deficiencies. They could also evaluate for illnesses that cause silent inflammation, which contributes to depression.

An enzyme is a protein that makes chemical reactions faster. Amylase is an enzyme produced by the pancreas and salivary glands. Ordering a test to measure the level of amylase in a client's blood can begin an investigation into whether the client has cancer of the tail of the pancreas.

Often, the first symptom of cancer of the tail of the pancreas is depression, and finding it then makes successful treatment more likely. You will not find it if you don't expect the unexpected. Having a high index of suspicion could save a life. That's an outcome that justifies being pushy.

When asking the treating physician to do an expensive test for a client, I feel more reluctant to be pushy, but Iris drove me to it out of desperation.

If you'd seen Iris, you wouldn't have noticed that she was a little pudgy. And you'd be puzzled by why, at thirty-eight, she still had noticeable acne.

At the first visit, she told me her biological clock stressed her out. She had stopped taking birth control pills over a year earlier. She and her husband got excited each time her period was late, only to realize it was just her irregular periods coming back—not a pregnancy.

Some days, Iris was so irritable during the sessions that I could say nothing right. Other times, she was pleasant but perplexed as she discussed how her seemingly random moodiness was wearing on her husband and girlfriends.

I thought about bipolar disorder II and character disorders as a cause of her irritability, but nothing seemed to fit. Then I noticed it—her faint mustache. I am troubled when I see additional facial hair on a female client because I know I must ask a question that I feel embarrassed to pose. I asked her anyway: "Do you have unwanted hair on parts of your body where you would not expect it?"

Iris did.

A sonogram and testosterone test later, polycystic ovarian syndrome was found to be the cause of her symptoms. Sometimes, tests are worth the cost.

Don't overlook toxic exposure or drink your pipes.

If you suspect that your client has been chronically exposed to toxins from work or living situations, you may want the doctor to test for heavy metals and other environmental and industrial toxins. According to Ecowatch (ecowatch.com), there are several environmental and industrial toxins. They include:

- Persistent organic pollutants (POPs), like dioxin
- Volatile organic compounds (VOCs)
- Phthalates
- Polybrominated diphenyl ethers (PBDEs)
- Polychlorinated biphenyls (PCBs)
- Polyfluoroalkyl substances (PFASs)
- Some metals, like lead, arsenic, copper, aluminum, cadmium, and mercury

Remember the phrase "mad as a hatter"? Many years ago, hat-making in England repeatedly exposed the people who made hats to mercury, which caused a toxic psychosis.

I also experienced toxic poisoning. A cistern fed water into my farmhouse. One day, a copper pipe burst. The plumber showed me where the acidity of the water from the cistern had eaten away the copper pipe. He told me we were drinking our pipes. That's when I realized that my diarrhea and abdominal pain were from copper toxicity.

The fellow who sold me the farm had built a new house on the hill that overlooked mine. When I told him about the copper in the pipes, he said he had not thought about it, but his stomach problems went away after he moved. A new water system solved the problem before we developed the mental symptoms that can also come from copper poisoning.

Perhaps the most common toxin people are exposed to, by themselves or others, is cigarette smoke. Clients may be reluctant to disclose to you or their health insurance company that they smoke for fear of having to pay more for their insurance.

Besides its toxic effect, smoking influences enzyme systems in the liver and alters how rapidly some medications are metabolized. Sometimes, a drug's level in the blood may be lower in smokers than in nonsmokers who are taking identical doses. If a client smokes, you may want to adjust their medication dose or pick another medication that is metabolized differently.

Chronic conditions sabotage progress.

Your client could be coping with multiple, long-standing, low-grade, chronic conditions that interfere with them fully working toward recovery. For example, untreated low back pain can impair sleep. As a result, your client is both tired and in pain as they attempt tasks. Addressing the pain becomes yet another arduous task.

Imagine a ditch-digger who has become tired because he is digging a ditch with his bare hands. He realizes that using the shovel he keeps in his truck would be easier, but he believes he can't spare the extra effort to get it.

Your client may have accepted their chronic illness as part of their daily life. They don't see how important it is to address their chronic illness as part of their progress. Show them how they are subtly undermining the hope and energy they need to mount a full-fledged effort to recover. By encouraging them to get treatment, you are suggesting a shovel.

Tiredness is a prevalent complaint.

It is not unusual for stressed or depressed clients to complain of tiredness among a collection of symptoms. Still, if tiredness is prominent in your client's presentation, think about anemia, malignancies, and, to a lesser extent, chronic fatigue syndrome. Rebekka Stadje et al. wrote an article that addresses the causes of tiredness: "The differential diagnosis of tiredness: A Systemic Review" (Stadje et al. 2016).

Include hepatitis and infectious diseases in your list of suspects, especially if your client is a world traveler.

Hypoxia can make life difficult and affect thinking.

When I was doing my rotation in pulmonary (lung) disease as a medical student, I admitted a woman who was unusually irritable and unpleasant to deal with. Doctors had already diagnosed her with an alpha-1 antitrypsin deficiency as the basis for her compromised lung function. When she was placed on oxygen, her entire personality seemed to shift. Her hypoxia (lack of oxygen) resolved, and she became delightful.

Suppose your client gives a multiyear history of significant cigarette smoking. Consider whether any of their irritability could come from some combination of vascular disease and chronic obstructive pulmonary disease (like emphysema). These might limit oxygen to their brain.

The experience and outcome of different surgeries can vary significantly.

Ask your client about the effect of a surgery on their mood and self-view. For example, suppose your client had surgery as a child. The experience might have included body image issues, opportunities to be bullied, missed sports and school, and early separation from parents. The environment could have felt unfriendly and unsafe. The parents might have subsequently become overprotective.

Perhaps your client had to deal with siblings who became jealous of the attention their parents showed your client. Other children might have made fun of their crutches, braces, or other devices.

Some surgeries have added emotional weight, like hysterectomies, mastectomies, orchiectomies, vasectomies, and tubal ligations.

In this chapter: I illustrated common and unusual explanations for what could happen to your client. Copper poisoning, hypoxia, pancreatic cancer, and PCOS are just uncommon enough to be overlooked. Tiredness is so common as to be hiding in plain sight.

In the next chapter: I deal with another difficulty so common that it's taken for granted. Everyone has difficulty sleeping from time to time. I cover the dangers of not getting the details of your client's sleep difficulties.

Chapter 7
Inquiring About Sleep

Adequate sleep is a cornerstone of treatment, and its absence is a clue to what is going wrong.

Know if your client gets a good night's sleep.

Sleep history is an integral part of the initial evaluation because good health requires an adequate amount of quality sleep. Glial cells are the brain's night janitors, and they work during deep sleep. If your client is not getting deep sleep, they won't feel rested. Inadequate sleep leads to impaired memory function the next day.

When your client is sleepless, is alone, lacks diversion, and has plenty of time to think, they can feel at the mercy of unwanted thoughts and suicidal thinking. Correcting insomnia can be a vital part of reducing suicidal risk.

Find out if your client takes naps during the day, as this can make it harder to fall asleep at night. Likewise, if they spend excessive time in bed over a twenty-four-hour period, they may not get concentrated sleep. If they sleep late in the morning, they may not be tired enough to fall asleep at night.

Some clients have schedules that don't allow them to be in bed long enough to get adequate sleep. Some work shifts disrupt the circadian rhythm. Do your clients have difficulty falling asleep, find that problems wake them up in the middle of the night, or wake up too early in the morning? Each pattern may mean something different.

Ask your clients if they have tried the cognitive-behavioral therapy program for insomnia (iCBT) or a sleep application. Do they use their computers or phones in nighttime mode to reduce blue light?

Clients who awaken in fright at a specific time may have been abused at that same time of night.

Sleep apnea can be lethal.

If anatomy creates obstructions to their breathing passages, even slender, young patients can have sleep apnea, which involves episodes of not breathing while sleeping. If your client is obese, there is even more reason to ask them about symptoms of sleep apnea. Because of how sleep apnea alters physiology, it is difficult for a client to lose weight if they have sleep apnea. As they gain weight, the obstructive structures get larger and obstruct more.

I once treated a middle-aged mother who had symptoms of sleep apnea and agreed to a sleep study. It revealed sleep apnea, but the insurance company did not feel it was bad enough for them to pay for a CPAP machine that would have provided continuous positive airway pressure. One night, my client died in her sleep.

Some symptoms, like tiredness, can be seen in various other illnesses. But still have a high index of suspicion to diagnose sleep apnea. It is a treatable condition that's worth keeping in mind.

While sleep difficulties often have a robust situational component, some are due to a primary sleep disorder. Still more are secondary to another illness. A history of sleep problems is a clue that your client might be depressed or anxious, or have a cyclic mood disorder.

Medication could be contributing to the sleep problem. Sometimes, the motor restlessness of ADHD continues into sleep as a sleep movement disorder. Older clients may have restless leg syndrome.

If a person drinks alcohol to fall asleep, they may find themselves awake and experiencing rebound symptoms when it wears off.

While sleep apps and iCBT may help some clients with sleep difficulties, it's important to look for sleep apnea and alcohol abuse because of their seriousness. Including a routine survey of sleep symptoms in your initial interview will help ensure that these essential questions are asked.

In this chapter: I looked at questions you might ask about sleep patterns and the need to consider sleep apnea in your history-taking.

In the next chapter: I take a brief first look at anxiety and panic, anxiety from physical causes like low blood sugar, and anxiety related to childhood experiences.

Chapter 8
Asking About Anxiety

There are different types of anxiety, and each may require a different approach. Physical factors cause some anxiety. Sometimes, panic-type anxiety reflects a lack of serotonin. Some kinds are situation-specific, and others are more generalized. Some anxiety is triggered by separation or feelings of being trapped. Children make assumptions about the world based on their experiences in the family, which may lead to feelings of anxiety and insecurity.

Quiz your client about which type of anxiety they might experience and its triggers.

When you ask your client about their anxiety, ask about any cluster of accompanying symptoms that might suggest hypoglycemia (low blood sugar), such as weakness, fast heart rate, shakiness, hunger, sweating, or tingling. How does the timing of symptoms fit with mealtimes?

Panic-type anxiety has a different intensity. When you see a client with panic symptoms, look for signs that indicate a need for medication that works on the serotonin system. Cramping, tingly fingers suggest that your client is hyperventilating during panic. I believe panic anxiety can occur at any time.

Ask if your client has tried a breath app to normalize their breathing, which helps reduce the fight-or-flight response. I wish breathing apps had been available in 2000. That year, my accountant told me I owed the Internal Revenue Service $64,000 in back taxes and penalties. It occurred to me that I could never pay it all back and the penalties would just mount. I had a full-blown panic attack.

I had two types of retirement plans. For several years, I had to pay for family health expenses and had not paid into the plan that required me to make annual contributions. I misinterpreted something I had been told and did not realize those contributions were compulsory. I consulted a tax lawyer, refiled multiple years of taxes, closed my second retirement account, and used the funds to pay off the reduced amount of $10,000 I owed. I was relieved, but for months, anything that looked like it came from the government triggered panic.

Ask your client about the situations in which they are anxious. Do they have anxiety only in social situations in which they could be embarrassed? Are they phobic?

Do your client's friends tell them, "If you don't have something to worry about, you find something"? If so, your client might have generalized anxiety disorder. This anxiety seems to be free-floating, as if being anxious is the person's default setting. It may come from the environment they grew up in. Children growing up in unsafe situations might logically assume that all situations are dangerous.

For example, imagine your family owned a McDonald's and you ate all your meals there. You would assume people ate on disposable dinnerware with plastic spoons because that is what you always did. It was all you knew. Now imagine your family owned a fancy French restaurant and you ate all your meals there. You would generalize your experience to think everyone ate with silverware and fancy plates on linen tablecloths.

As I interview a client, I try to imagine them as a child and ask myself what environment surrounded them. I aim to grasp their logical assumptions about that environment and how those assumptions would, in turn, lead to insecurity or encourage other behaviors.

For example, if a client's mother had an alcohol use disorder, the client might assume people are well-intentioned but undependable and unpredictable. They may struggle to rely on others and be uncertain about people's ability to keep their promises. They might have learned to be cautious about what they say to their mother to avoid angering her. They would logically assume that sharing their thoughts with others leads to adverse outcomes.

I listen for evidence that confirms or challenges my notion about a source of the anxiety. I remind myself that my confirmation bias would cause me to favor information that confirms my beliefs. Then, I try to pursue different ideas more fully.

There are many avenues to explore in taking a client history because there are so many situations and life events that could be behind anxiety:

- Abandonment anxiety, for example, suggests that your client has been affected by losses when people died, moved away, or rejected them.
- Did their environment make them want to escape the situation? Could it have left them continually anxious about getting trapped with a partner or a job they don't like?
- Might they have grown up in a repressive environment that generated unacceptable anger and fear of punishment for nonadherence?
- Are they anxious about experiencing retribution for guilty thoughts related to their situation?
- Does your client feel unprepared for a test they are taking or need to do a job they are not qualified to do?

In this chapter: I covered panic-type anxiety and anxiety from low blood sugar. I noted how childhood situations can lead to later anxiety and alluded to other types of anxiety that we'll touch on later.

In the next chapter: These first chapters have concerned themselves with gathering information about more current aspects of a client's situation. Now the discussion shifts to a more detailed examination of their past. Next, we explore questions about the role of various factors in early client development and family function, including early trauma, delayed milestones, familial diseases, birth order, family tragedy, and the nature of the family system.

Chapter 9

Discovering Developmental and Family Histories

It's important to know about maternal events, genetics, birth order, and family dynamics.

Family members can tell you about developmental milestones, bonding issues, and trauma that occurred when the client was too young to know about it.

Sometimes, a child's name reflects a family's expectations of them. There may be a clue in their name to their task of replacing a deceased person or exemplifying a particular quality that their parents value.

Intensive care unit (ICU) nurses impress me with their consistent efforts to provide human touch to infants under their care. I suspect it makes a difference. But I still worry about clients who spent their first few days or weeks in the ICU because being separated from the mother can impact the mother-child bond. Oxytocin, a hormone that a mother's brain secretes in the postpartum period, motivates her to bond with her newborn. I worry about a mother's oxytocin level going back to pre-pregnancy levels before the infant can get out of the ICU and go home. Of course, oxytocin is just one factor in a mother's ability to bond with her infant. Most parents take every chance to visit and hold their infant in the hospital.

Still, clients who start their lives in the ICU may have the early impression that the environment is hurtful, with people having to do necessary procedures on their bodies. Sometimes, prematurity can be associated with anxiety-producing respiratory distress.

It can be challenging to learn about developmental milestones. Your client could have been too young to register them, and parents may not recall them. You might ask a general question about whether a client mastered a task early or their parents told them they lagged behind their siblings. That could lead to more specific information about when they crawled, walked, talked, read, and met other developmental milestones. This information may provide insight into their brain development and early success.

Trauma at a particular developmental stage affects a child's ability to master the tasks of that stage. So, knowing when the trauma happened is essential. For example:

- Did the trauma occur when the client was developing object constancy, being toilet trained, experiencing oedipal issues, etc.?
- Did the parents witness a regression in development at those times?

- Could the client have had a childhood illness that required hospitalization and separated them from their parents?
- Not all trauma is emotional. Perhaps your client sustained a concussion from a fall or accident as a child.

In today's world, it is often necessary for both parents to work, and neither one may have maternity or paternity leave that allows them to stay home for a long period after a child's birth. Both parents play an essential role in a child's development and in supporting the other partner. Sometimes, an extended family member saves the day by providing childcare. When I see a client who thrived despite early parental separation, I ask about grandparents' involvement.

A clue to your adult client's separation issues might be how they reacted to going off to school.

Clues hide in the complex web of family history.

The family history piece of the initial interview usually includes demographic data about family members, including ages, occupations, and living situations. It can get complicated quickly, with blended families, stepparents, half-siblings, stepsiblings, and adopted members. Often, grandparents, aunts, and uncles play essential roles as well.

Eleanor's case illustrates how the difference in age between your client and their parents can sometimes give you a clue about dynamics.

Eleanor, my last client of the day, was a twenty-one-year-old college senior who was neatly dressed in a student nurse's uniform that still showed signs of having been ironed the night before. She looked, for all the world, like the kind of girl every mother wishes her son would bring home to dinner.

She immediately apologized for being late and thanked me for extending my day to make room for her. I explained that I understood that student nurses on their clinical rotations had little control over when their mentor let them go. I told her that I usually made time later in my day for them. Within the first twenty minutes, she apologized four times for things she couldn't control.

Since freshman year, she had lived with two girls who had known each other since grade school. She felt like a third wheel. Then she met a young political science major who was a great guy. They developed a serious relationship, which went smoothly until a pregnancy scare brought up their differences about having children. He wanted them. She didn't. Eleanor was considering a tubal ligation.

Things were up in the air, too, about their future job and schooling plans. If Eleanor and her boyfriend were going to be in the same town the next year, they would have to coordinate her job location with where he went to graduate school. Eleanor wondered if children would be a deal-breaker.

She talked enthusiastically about how much she wanted to work in pediatrics with special-needs children who might feel left out of the usual childhood activities. She told me that her mom had halted her own teaching career after Eleanor's twin sisters were born and had just gotten back into teaching when she became pregnant with Eleanor. My client felt terrible that her mom, who had chronic back pain, had more years to work before she could retire. She was determined not to become her mother.

Eleanor's life's theme emerged as therapy progressed. Her twin sisters, just like her roommates, had a bond with one another that she was not part of. Eleanor was an extra and felt like a burden. She'd picked up on her mom's resentment at having an extra baby later in life. Feeling apologetic for being born, she had spent her life trying to make up for it by being a dutiful child and an excellent student. She believed that God forgave sins. But somehow, she felt God could not forgive *her* sins. She recalled how, during Communion, she feared the wafers and wine would run out before the priest got to her.

In therapy, she struggled with self-possession and the difference between what was her responsibility and what was her mother's. The first clue to the dynamic was how old her mother was when Eleanor was born.

Family histories may reflect cherished family myths, overgeneralizations, and fears that disclosing secrets may result in disloyalty or loss of personal safety.

When hearing about significant family life events, remember that there is the event, and then there is what the family members tell themselves about its meaning. The ascribed meaning may have a bigger effect. For example, family members explain that a client's brother drank excessively because he was fired from a good job without justification. Later, you learn he had been drinking excessively since high school.

Clients' descriptions of their family members often sound like overgeneralizations or cultural stereotypes. My ears perk up when I hear clients idealize or vilify family members. I wonder where the supporting evidence is.

Your client may feel disloyal about revealing family secrets. A more accurate picture of the family may emerge over later sessions, when they are more comfortable with you.

Revealing family secrets can be dangerous. I remember a young woman I treated in a residential setting who said she would not talk about her family because they were in organized crime. She made some progress in her recovery, but she never spoke about her family life. I was convinced that she was putting me on with her story. But then a big black limousine with tinted windows pulled up when she was discharged. The fellow who got out could have come right out of *The Sopranos*.

Family genetics are important determinants in planning treatment.

When your client speaks about a family history of mental illness and addiction, be aware that secrets may have been kept from them as a child. Their information may be distorted or incomplete.

Have them explain the symptoms they saw in their family member. Did a doctor make the relative's diagnosis after an adequate evaluation? Keep in mind that the doctor could have made a mistake.

Unthinking clients may quickly label unlikable relatives as hysterical, borderline, bipolar, sociopathic, or narcissistic without adequate evidence.

An accurate psychiatric history of a client's family is vital because of the genetic risk to the client. For example, suppose I have a client whose parent has been clearly diagnosed with bipolar disorder. In that case, I will have a higher index of suspicion that my client has latent bipolar disorder, and I will avoid medications that could spark mania.

Clients with bipolar disorder in their family may be worried about also having a bipolar disorder. Help them understand that not everyone at higher risk develops the disease.

Birth order may have implications
for your client's experiences.

If your client is the firstborn with several siblings, ask if the older siblings were given responsibility for raising the younger siblings. Would the younger sibs resent them for setting limits on them or perhaps see them as the actual parent?

Remember that the firstborn was "his or her majesty the baby" until the second-born came along. The firstborn may experience narcissistic rage (intense anger triggered by threats to a self-centered person's self-esteem) toward siblings for displacing them. I remember a firstborn asking their parents, "Wasn't I enough?"

The firstborn may be the icebreaker who struggles with the parents and was denied certain privileges. As time passes, the parents become less uptight and give the subsequent children those same privileges. Did the firstborn develop envy if they had fewer opportunities than subsequent siblings who benefited from the family's improving financial condition?

Was the firstborn child planned? Did pregnancy result in an unintended marriage? Did the parents have them (or adopt them) in hopes of saving a foundering relationship? If the parents are much older than the client, was the client an unexpected, late-life baby? Were the client's older parents too tired to keep up with them, or did they repeatedly set limits?

The baby in the family may feel underestimated or need to prove themselves in the face of successful older siblings. Were they expected to stay home so there would be no empty nest?

Ask who made a difference in your client's life.

Imagine a plant in dry soil that sends roots to other areas for water. Children are like plants that reach out to grandparents, aunts, uncles, friends, and neighbors for affection when the nuclear family garden is dry. When you hear about a dry family garden, look for the grandmother whose eyes lit up when your client came into the room and who showed them they were loved. Ask about the coach or teacher who made a difference in your client's life. Also, remember that sexual perpetrators of all ages look for the needy child like a wolf noticing a straggling sheep.

Understandably, a parent who loses their spouse is grief-stricken and preoccupied with the loss. Did a client who lost a parent feel like, at least for a time, they lost both parents? This situation pushes siblings closer, as often happens, too, with children of dysfunctional parents.

Consider your client's family system.

Does your client come from a patriarchal or matriarchal culture? Is the family hierarchy disordered, resulting in the child being forced to operate on a parental level?

Is the family system the stereotypical enmeshed system, where parents get upset if the child doesn't eat their vegetables? Did your client, as a result, develop discipline from their parents' rules? Are they now unable to think for themselves?

Could the family system be the stereotypically disengaged family, where members do their own thing and don't get upset until they hear that a child has been arrested? In this system, the child may be an original thinker without self-discipline.

Perhaps it's a mixture of the two types of systems.

Is there a family history of parents undergoing the uncoupling process over the years? Does one parent experience their relationship with their partner as uncomfortable? Are they then triangulating in their job, hobby, or another relationship to regulate the distance between themselves and their partner? Your client may have grown up as these processes were unfolding.

In this chapter: We discussed how family events, family systems, developmental issues, birth order, and parental age have affected your client.

In the next chapter: I examine the client's relationship history and introduce the processes of uncoupling, generational projection, and mythmaking, which your questions may uncover. Being a military dependent, having social anxiety, and having ADHD are mentioned as shaping relationships. The first breakup is highlighted as a risk for suicide.

Chapter 10
Exploring the
Relationship History

Your clients may choose partners who are like their parents. Some clients pull a third party into a relationship to create a more comfortable distance. Others select a partner or friend whose personality naturally leads to conflicts similar to the client's past relationships. Skillful questioning can uncover patterns in the uncoupling of relationships and the myths clients use to explain their dissolution.

Identify patterns in your client's relationships.

Ask yourself the following questions about your client to identify patterns:

- Are they comfortable in their own skin, have a clearly defined sense of who they are, and seek friends and partners with similar maturity levels without feeling intimidated?

- In friendships, do they do things without always expecting to be rewarded?
- Would you describe their relationships as directed toward mutual benefits rather than emotional connectedness?
- Are they too detached or too clingy in relationships?
- Do they manipulate their friends?
- Can they make friends only with people who are just like them?
- Are they frequent victims?
- Have they set up masochistic relationships in which they sadistically induce guilt in people they allow to take advantage of them?
- Are they uncomfortable in one-on-one relationships and feel the need to bring a third person into the relationship to have distance?
- Do they exhibit an approach-avoidance conflict in getting the relationship they want? In that case, they want closeness and simultaneously want to avoid rejection.
- Do they fear something bad will happen if they have a successful relationship because they have gotten what they desire?
- Do they sabotage a relationship that is going well because they believe it can't last?

In looking at friendships, ask your client if they frequently moved around growing up. Some clients had parents whose jobs, such as the military, required them to move frequently. Your client may have developed social skills to make quick friends but didn't get the chance to have lifelong friendships because of the moves.

It is easy to offend clients when asking them about their romantic relationships.

Your clients may be in relationships of various kinds, including committed, uncommitted, hookups, asexual, and friends with benefits. It is best to let a client tell you about their sex, gender, and sexual orientation rather than making assumptions. Make a general statement showing your willingness to listen to any of their concerns about these areas. That will show your client that you are open to talking about their relationship.

They may feel you are ignoring the nature of their relationship as you try to understand their romantic relationships from a clinical perspective. They may wonder if you are confusing matters of the heart with matters of the brain. Be sensitive to your client's need for privacy. After getting to know and trust you, they will likely feel more comfortable being open.

If your client tells you they had to drink alcohol to diminish anxiety before socializing, suspect that they have social anxiety disorder. Some clients are just lucky to find that their first date is the love of their life. Clients with social anxiety may dread dating and settle for Mr. He'll Do instead of Mr. Right. The prospect of divorcing and having to date again may cause them to stay in a loveless marriage.

If you get a sense that your client is impulsive in their relationships, ask yourself if they could have manic episodes, ADHD, or a problem with substance abuse.

Your client might reasonably expect that sexual behavior is affectionate. If your questions reveal compulsive sexual behavior, besides looking for other addictions, look for evidence that your client grew up in a setting that would lead to them being desperate for even a moment of feeling wanted and cared about.

Look for behavioral patterns as you ask clients about their past significant relationships, how long they lasted, and why they ended. For example, do you see them reject agreeable partners in favor of a partner who is distant like their parent? Because clients sometimes seek out partners who are like their parents and grandparents.

Jessie, age twenty-three and wearing a soft brown corduroy shirt and Levi's jeans, looked like he could pull out a guitar at any moment and play a gentle love song. He'd grown up watching his dad lose arguments with his mother. Jessie wanted his dad to stand up for himself and saw his willingness to compromise as a weakness. His dad's interest in keeping the peace in the face of his mother's demands made it hard for Jessie to identify with him.

Jessie was personable and attracted women who found that his easy nature spoke to their wish to be nurtured. He made friends with these women, but he was attracted to opinionated, spunky, assertive women. They were more like his dad's mother, who had run the construction business she'd inherited. She'd had a firm hand that commanded the respect of the men who worked for her. Yet Jesse struggled to assert himself with the women he was attracted to, just like his father and grandfather struggled in their relationships with strong women.

In therapy, he could see that this pattern spanned generations. He came to recognize when compromise made sense and learned to assert himself more appropriately while still relishing the company of women who were independent thinkers.

Breakups are consequential
and often not what they seem.

Some clients marry the first person they date, while everyone else walking down the aisle broke up with everyone they dated before they met their partner. Breakups are commonplace. Overlooking how consequential the first one is for your client can cause you to miss a potentially vital piece of information.

I did consultations in a general hospital that required all patients who had been in the intensive care unit (ICU) after a suicide attempt to see a psychiatrist before they could be discharged. I was surprised by how many of these patients experienced their first breakup shortly before their attempt.

Some of these patients had loved with the abandon that comes from never having been hurt before. They often talked about how the rejection deeply disturbed their self-perception and self-worth. It seemed impossible for them to imagine a future without their beloved, and they experienced an unbearable emotional state of frantic hopelessness.

Oddly, on rare occasions, surviving the suicide attempt seemed like a rebirth. The patient felt they had survived for a reason and could start over. While the vast majority of people are not suicidal after their first breakup, the first breakup is always significant.

Fortunately, not all relationships end in breakups. Discovering how your client solved everyday problems to maintain ties tells you something about their ability to tolerate frustration, be flexible, and find mutually agreeable solutions.

Maintaining a relationship calls on problem-solving skills, as does the process of ending a relationship.

In her book *Uncoupling: Turning Points in Intimate Relationships,* Diane Vaughn describes how uncoupling is a gradual process, as one partner develops a personal and social identity apart from their partner. As you listen to descriptions of breakups, realize that the uncoupling process can take a long time. For example, let's say a client tells you they divorced their partner because the partner was having an affair. But the affair might have been a reaction to your client's prolonged distancing behavior. In that case, your client was the first one to be dissatisfied (Vaughan 1990).

Peter Weiss, in his book *Marital Separation,* talks about how people construct a myth to explain to themselves why the separation occurred. The myth helps the individual get their head around it. Years later, they realize that the myth did not tell the entire story. I have had clients agree with this idea. As you listen to your clients discuss breakups, ask yourself about their myth and how it has helped them recover from the loss (Weiss 1975).

In this chapter: I offered questions you can ask to uncover patterns in relationships. You were introduced to the idea of uncoupling and mythmaking.

In the next chapter: I discuss the multiple fields your client has had to function in. Asking questions about their track record helps you predict their future behavior.

Chapter 11

Finding Evidence of How Your Client Functions in Different Settings

School history, job history, substance abuse history, military history, and legal history give you clues about how well your client has functioned in different settings. A review of systems gathers symptoms that your other histories may have missed.

Past school challenges reveal clients' coping skills and deficits.

Did your client have trouble leaving home to start school? When they had academic or social difficulties, what was also happening in their life at that time?

If they were home-schooled, why were they? What opportunities for socialization were provided to them in their school situation and outside school?

Did a later birthdate put them developmentally behind their classmates in competitions? Were they in the school band or on the sports team? Being part of a working group suggests they can work with others, follow directions, and persist in tasks. These abilities reflect a client's ego strength and executive function.

Ask about other evidence of their strengths, like their grades, how far they went in school, and what they had to push through to get there. How did they deal with failures? Did they have to work their way through school? If they were in a fraternity or sorority, were they in a leadership position? How did they handle their fraternity's or sorority's compulsory social events?

How did they cope with stressors? Did they have to deal with a bully or transfer midyear? Were they a first-generation college student? How did they cope with diversity? Were they in a minority group? Did they experience discrimination or microaggression? Were they sexually assaulted?

Listen for evidence that might suggest they have ADHD. For more on this, go to my YouTube video *Disastrous Fallacies about ADHD*. https://www.youtube.com/watch?v=V3V9sjIwyEI

Besides revealing strengths, the job history opens a window into a client's values.

What an opportunity you get to discover new worlds when you take the job history! I have worked with a diverse range of clients, including shrimpers, soldiers, exotic dancers, bookies, prisoners, correctional officers, cooks, American seamen, professors, chicken factory workers, drug dealers, nurses, test pilots, snipers, and others whose worlds I might otherwise not have known. Your clients will also enrich your life as you learn from the relative comfort of your office chair.

My clients in the poultry industry taught me about the excitement when a truck dropped off hundreds of "eggs with legs" to be cared for. They described being so careful that their chicks did not overheat in the summer or get too cold in the winter. They were as vigilant as a mother hen. They oversaw every aspect of their chicks' well-being, providing the right amount of the proper feed, clean water, and sanitary conditions. They talked about the joy of watching their chicks grow. After months of care, they faced the sadness of seeing the truck come and take their charges away. They had to content themselves with the idea that they had given their chickens a healthy life despite its brevity.

I listened to them discuss the pressure to upgrade facilities and their concern that failing to do so would result in losing their contract, which would require them to go into significant debt.

I also got to know the workers at the plant who caught the chickens. I saw where the chickens had scarred their hands when they'd held multiple chickens simultaneously with the chickens' claws between their fingers.

I met with plant workers who showed me their fingers with arthritis caused by repeatedly processing chicken under cold conditions and performing the same movements.

After working with poultry industry clients, I appreciate the care and sacrifice that goes into the chicken I eat.

Your questions about work will resemble the ones you asked about school. Each situation allows your client to show their ability to compromise, delay gratification, be flexible, and tolerate frustration. They also reveal the elements of ego strength. Work requires effort and the ability to understand and follow orders.

Ask your client how long they worked at each job and why they left. How did they get along with their bosses? Were they sexually harassed or abused? Did they show leadership? How did they relate to their coworkers?

In asking about jobs, you can touch on their goals and where they find meaning. Their answers to these first questions may allow you to broach the subject of their values and the role their spiritual beliefs play in their life.

Unmanageability is a hallmark of addiction to alcohol and other drugs.

Look for signs of intoxication and withdrawal, which may suggest your client has a problem with drugs or alcohol. Chronic marijuana use can cause clients to be unusually forgetful in answering the mental status questions and generally too relaxed and laid back in the interview, given their situation.

You will find an explanation of how to take an alcohol history on the MedSchool website about alcohol history-taking: https://medschool.co/history/basics/alcohol-history-taking

The Foundations of Clinical Medicine of the University of Washington discusses how to take a substance use history here: https://uw.pressbooks.pub/fcmtextbook/chapter/substance-use-history/

There may be characteristic gaps in an alcoholic's history because they have had blackouts and memory gaps.

Sometimes, they are in recovery, and they wonder why their family is not recovering as quickly. It may be because of things the alcoholic doesn't remember doing.

Getting a history from someone who is actively addicted involves asking for information from the brain of a person whose memory is impaired. Recovering from addiction is more complicated because the brain that is trying to recover is the same brain that is impaired. Collateral information becomes even more critical. According to AA (Alcoholics Anonymous), alcoholics get into recovery by developing honesty, openness, and willingness. The lack of these qualities when they meet you makes history-taking unreliable.

Clients may resume drinking or using substances while in treatment. Relapse is a process that may start long before usage resumes. Make asking about the signs of relapse and resumption of use a part of your ongoing treatment routine.

The biggest diagnostic clue that a client is addicted is that their life is unmanageable. Because of this, starting treatment in an outpatient setting that is not an intensive outpatient program may be less effective. You may find questions about how abuse has made life unmanageable more meaningful to your client than simply asking how much or how often they consume.

Years ago, I took part in an organization called The Chemical People, which Nancy Reagan sponsored. We surveyed students K–12. We found that one in ten students had someone in their household who drank an unspecified amount of alcohol daily. It was not clear how people who drank limited amounts of alcohol exaggerated the numbers, but it still seemed like an unusual finding.

We were sure we had made a mistake in our surveying procedure. Then we learned that other groups were finding the same thing. While this finding may be exaggerated, I have since had a higher index of suspicion that some of my clients were adult children of alcoholics (ACOAs).

Several books in this book's bibliography address the treatment of ACOAs. More about this heterogeneous group will be mentioned later.

There are hidden traumas in serving our country in the military.

The line of questioning about military history will be similar to asking about job history. But with military clients, you're also looking for a history of risk factors for post-traumatic stress disorder (PTSD) from combat. Learn about separations from the family, financial hardships associated with service, and how your client adapted to civilian life. You may find that attending the Advanced Individual Training School of their choice shaped the rest of their military experience.

A person may not have been in the military but may have lived in a war-torn area, be in law enforcement, or be in other situations that put their life at risk.

One of my clients had all the symptoms of PTSD but no obvious source of trauma. Then he explained that his family made moonshine liquor. He'd grown up in the woods in a house surrounded by booby traps and alarms. His family was always on guard for trespassers and federal law enforcement officers who would destroy their still. He had lived for years with the constant threat of violence.

Implausible explanations and gaps in your client's timeline suggest legal difficulties.

Antisocial behavior is not the only way clients get into legal trouble. Legal troubles may be a clue to a past episode of mania, psychosis, or substance abuse. It may suggest a problem with impulse control or judgment. You may find that your client is not forthcoming in answering your questions about legal entanglements. You may be alerted to possible legal difficulties by gaps in your client's timeline or ways others have treated them that make little sense without knowing their undisclosed legal problems.

If a history suggests that your client has an antisocial personality disorder, you may get some further clues by giving them the Disgust Scale. You might enjoy *That's Disgusting: Unraveling the Mysteries of Repulsion* by Rachel Hertz (2012).

The *Review of Systems* may catch things you have missed.

The questionnaire I use asks clients about the common symptoms of depression, anxiety disorders, bipolar disorders, social anxiety, suicidal thinking, obsessions, and psychosis. I follow up on their responses during the interview. Sometimes, clients endorse everything as a cry for help.

Familiarize yourself with the typical symptoms of these common mental disorders. This book assumes you already have this foundation of knowledge, which helps you understand the many clients whose presentations are not baffling and more easily fit into diagnostic categories. Review them in the *Diagnostic and Statistical Manual V*. The Cleveland Clinic discusses the DSM-5 here: https://my.

clevelandclinic.org/health/articles/24291-diagnostic-and-statistical-manual-dsm-5

You may want to use one of these diagnostic instruments to clarify your diagnosis further:

- The Yale-Brown Obsessive Compulsive Scale (YBOCS)
- The Young Mania Rating Scale, The 21-item Hypomania Checklist
- The Montgomery Asberg Depression Rating Scale (MADRS).

In this chapter: I dealt with past client function as predictive of your client's future.

In the next chapter: We will shift back to the here and now and look at the objective evidence of your client's function.

Chapter 12

Evaluating a Client's Mental Status

An effective mental status evaluation helps determine the risk of mania, psychosis, and suicide. Odd client presentations and out-of-date techniques may lead to mistakes.

Thoroughly document your client's mental status to avoid a disastrous surprise later.

Unlike history, which is a subjective record, the mental status exam includes objective signs of dysfunction. Your observations of your client's appearance begin your examination of their mental status. Most clients will have essentially normal mental status exams. Their ability to answer your history questions and their ordinary behavior during the interview often assure you they are intelligent and in touch with reality. That makes the mental status exam seem like a waste of time.

When I reviewed medical records to help insurance companies decide whether a client was disabled, I found that psychologists, with their particular training, were the best at documenting mental status. Other providers were not as consistent.

When your client remarks that they are forgetful, you rarely feel you have to doubt them or measure how forgetful they are. Insurance companies are not satisfied with the client's claim that they have cognitive problems. Insurance companies want to read objective evidence. The lack of an adequate mental status exam could cost your client coverage.

When you create records, you have no way of knowing how they will be used later. While confidentiality is the rule, clients may waive that in different situations, giving insurance companies and other organizations access for billing and other reasons.

Your records may be consulted in evaluating a client's competence to cooperate with their lawyer at trial. Part of an evaluation for guardianship for an older person suspected of having dementia might involve your records. A malpractice attorney may review your records for objective evidence to support your actions. Clients who later seek custody or apply for security clearance may have to rely on your records.

Some things a client tells you do not contribute to their treatment, are embarrassing, and can be left out without being detrimental to a clear understanding of their case. It would be beneficial to understand what information must be disclosed in the courtroom regarding a client session.

Serial mental status exams help determine whether your treatment is working and can provide guidance for future decisions about medication and therapy.

When a history is challenging to take, it can be a clue to the changes in mental status seen in psychotic, manic, and suicidal clients.

Evaluating mental status is most crucial in deciding suicidal risk, violence risk, and the presence of psychosis or mania. Jeffrey P. Kahn and Andre Barciela Veras, in their March 2022 article in *Current Psychiatry,* proposed different subtypes of psychosis and identified early mental status changes to help you identify psychosis early: https://www.mdedge.com/psychiatry/article/252208/schizophrenia-other-psychotic-disorders/psychoses-5-comorbidity-defined/page/0/4

Psychosis is a disease process that is actively destructive to the brain, and early treatment can make a big difference in long-term prognosis.

A change in cognitive ability might be one of only a few clues to a serious situation, like a brain tumor, schizophrenia, or severe depression.

Think about schizophrenia when your client has problems recognizing what people around them are feeling, appears forgetful, can't stay on the subject, thinks too slowly, and can't reason well. Cognitive deficits may precede the more obvious positive symptoms of schizophrenia.

You may see depressed clients who have a good deal of personal strength. They continue to function for years as their depression worsens. They are successful people who don't seem to be in trouble. However, their depression has transformed into difficulty with intrusive, dark thoughts that border on delusions about the hopelessness of their situation. They may have high lethality because they don't show that they are intensely miserable and have suicidal thoughts that they feel embarrassed to admit. They don't tell you about it, but subtle changes in their cognitive ability can alert you if you are looking for them.

Look for a narrowing of thinking in suicidal clients. For example, they see no way to please an important person or feel okay without that person's approval. Being anything less than perfect is unimaginable. They can't envision getting past the loss of a loved one. It seems reasonable to them to assume their problem is permanent and permeates their entire life. Is there an absence of protective factors? Is their anhedonia severe?

When a client voices delusional ideas or responds to voices or visual hallucinations, it is easier to define their abnormal mental status because the changes are less subtle. Other changes are more nuanced and challenging to identify.

Sometimes, the first clue to an abnormal mental status is that the history is difficult to obtain. At first, a client may seem to be taking extra time to respond thoughtfully to your questions. Later, it becomes clear that their thought processing speed is abnormally slow.

You may work excessively hard to get a timeline for what happened and realize their speech is circumstantial and poorly organized. When asked a question, they get distracted by something else, and it appears they have problems sustaining attention or are perhaps distracted by auditory hallucinations.

They speak too fast, and it is difficult to follow their pressured speech. You cannot follow their logic and realize they have a loose associational trend.

After you've made repeated efforts to get more details about past events, it is clear that their long-term memory is poor. When you must repeatedly oversimplify what you are telling them, it's a clue that they may think concretely or have a limited fund of information, vocabulary, or education.

When you feel these frustrations, document what you notice. Tell them a story, like the ones in the Wechsler Logical Memory Test, to look at short-term memory. Ask about their ability to follow a movie. Ask them to recall a phone number you gave them. You may want to do a more formal test of their digit recall to test working memory.

I sometimes have a client read a short passage about the causes of World War II. I want to see how well they can keep the various causes in their mind and summarize what they read as a measure of reading comprehension.

I might ask a family member how often the client forgets to buy items when they go grocery shopping. You may be surprised that a client with an excellent fund of acquired knowledge has trouble doing your mental status exam's simple tasks.

Your client may have a specific math or language problem that results in mistakes on tests of cognitive ability, and their lower score may not accurately reflect their overall function.

Dr Ziad Nasreddine of Moca Cognition invented the Montreal Test of Cognitive Ability (MOCA), which is helpful when you have questions about your client's cognition. (https://www. mocacognition.com/the-moca-test/)

Dr. Marshal Folstein and Dr. Susan Folstein created the Mini-Mental State Exam (MMSE) (https://meded.temertymedicine. utoronto.ca/sites/default/files/assets/resource/document/ mini-mental-state-examinationmmse.pdf), as another standardized screening instrument.

Client presentations can be misleading.

Sometimes, manic patients have an infectious mood, and I feel entertained during the interview. I must catch myself and realize that the reality they are blithely describing is dire. Their affect is inappropriate for the content of their speech. The soundtrack does not fit the picture.

Other times, a client's eloquent description of the source of their despair might mislead me and make me feel that it is logical to feel that way. The description was an intellectualization to justify the depressive, dark view that came from the client's significant depression. The depression came first, and the client developed a framework to explain it to themselves.

A client may present a very logical but incorrect argument for why they feel a certain way. A wife once gave me multiple plausible reasons for why she no longer desired her husband. After her gynecologist placed her on oral testosterone, she returned to tell me she did not care whether her husband helped with chores; she desired him. She realized she had constructed an explanation for something that actually had a physical cause. An articulate, depressed person may do the same thing to explain the biological process of being depressed.

False deficits can come from asking questions that don't consider your client's background. Don't ask a city dweller who has never been on a farm what it means when people say, "Make hay while the sun shines." If you test your client's abstracting ability using proverbial sayings, pick a modern one that is common to their culture. In getting a history, you will have already found evidence of the client's ability to abstract and make judgments.

Does your client's lack of emotional modulation make you feel on edge? Do you hear your client vilify or idealize the people in their history? That may suggest they do all-or-none thinking. Your reactions and feelings can be another instrument in evaluating your client's mental status.

***

In this chapter: I warned of the hazards of not incorporating a mental status examination into your routine. I also pointed out how a mental status evaluation can help you make critical decisions about suicidal risk, violence risk, mania, and psychosis. We covered how you can use your own feelings as a tool of observation.

In the next chapter: I shift toward the future by discussing elements of the treatment plan. We will look at the necessity of keeping an open mind and collaborating with your client to create an individualized treatment plan that may involve multiple providers.

Chapter 13

Formulating Dynamics and Agreeing on a Treatment Plan

Flexibility, collaboration, and open-mindedness make for better treatment planning.

A dynamic formulation hypothesizes how the client thinks.

In the dynamic formulation, ideas about the dynamics that go into the client's difficulties are briefly summarized. I will write more about dynamics in a later chapter.

Making a diagnosis is the most dangerous thing a therapist does.

Making the diagnosis can cause you to close your mind to other possibilities, especially to the possibility of a stroke. Consider the diagnosis a working one. You can change it as you get more information, which may be contradictory. Even the *Diagnostic and Statistical Manual* is continually being debated and revised. The scientific nature of our practice fosters a constant search for a better explanation of what we observe.

On rare occasions, symptoms could be a disease process that is not yet defined. Perhaps a client has a disease that occurs so rarely that little is known about it. Keeping an open mind means being okay with uncertainty. It's natural to discount what the client tells you when it doesn't fit what you have been taught. When the situation safely allows, consider delaying diagnosis to get more input. Discuss findings with colleagues. In this way, you guard against confirmation bias.

Remember the growth mindset that views clients as continually growing, changing, and learning from experience. The growth mindset particularly applies to children and adolescents. The electronic medical record funnels data into preset choices. Remember that you are looking at the client at one point and that you have an incomplete picture with possibly inaccurate information.

Insurance companies want diagnoses. I am caught between wanting to be precise and document the level of dysfunction with what would be a more serious diagnosis and knowing that people, especially young people, are continually growing and changing. The data may also be incomplete or misleading. I know my diagnosis is a working diagnosis that applies at a point in time, but the insurance company employees looking at the database may not appreciate that.

Treatment planning is a collaborative effort and may include a referral.

As you construct the treatment plan with your client's help, remember that change takes effort. General health measures, like exercise, proper diet, and time in the sunlight, help your client be healthy enough to do the work.

As you begin collaborating with your client, ask them if they want your opinion and suggestions. Asking permission shows respect and your awareness that what they expect from therapy may differ.

When surveying your client's strengths and weaknesses, look at their support system and finances. Your treatment plan may include referrals to address different physical problems. You may need to recruit multiple providers who team with each other, each collaborating on separate elements of your client's treatment.

It would be easy to discount the role of antidepressants in helping your depressed clients because antidepressants have traditionally taken a long time to work, have aggravating side effects, and may not have resulted in significant improvement. Now there are new antidepressants with different mechanisms of action that work rapidly and more effectively, with significantly fewer side effects. Auvelity and Spravato are just two examples. These advances support therapeutic optimism and a referral to a prescriber for clients who feel depressed.

The plan could involve referring clients out because of a conflict of interest. I once listened to a woman complain about her unfaithful husband and then realized that I was also treating the woman her husband was seeing. Occasionally, you may know you are not a good match for a patient.

Perhaps they should see someone with a unique skill set because of a particular type of problem they have. Clients may need psychological testing, drug testing, or neurological evaluation. Consider the benefits of group therapy.

In this chapter: I emphasized keeping an open mind as you collaborate with your client and other providers to establish a diagnosis and the plan of action that follows from it. Like the diagnosis, the treatment plan is a working concept that can change with new ideas and situations.

In the next chapter: We examine how therapy may impact you. Isolated, anxious, doubtful, vulnerable, phony, and heroic are just some of the many ways therapists feel. They count on their clients' grace and teachers' wisdom as they gain experience and eventual quiet satisfaction in doing effective therapy.

Part 2

UNDERSTANDING THE THERAPEUTIC RELATIONSHIP BY INTEGRATING WHAT YOU HAVE LEARNED

Clues about who your client is and the potential for an effective therapeutic relationship come from various sources. This section helps you as you formulate these clues, gathered in part from your early observations and the client history.

This incubating phase of therapy, which is more reflective, feels like a needed step. Integrating these clues will help you decide how to proceed with treatment.

Your more immediate hints may come from noticing how your client affects you and seeing the emergence of transference and countertransference in the therapeutic relationship. It may become apparent how culture and upbringing affected them in specific ways. Other evidence will come from their dynamics, their type of character, and how they react to events in therapy and life situations.

This section—along with Part 3, which discusses client dynamics—lays the groundwork for Part 4, which discusses how to do therapy.

Chapter 14

Therapists' Experience of Providing Therapy

While usually a source of quiet satisfaction, providing therapy may also lead to a range of emotions, including doubt, fear, surprise, pride, and loneliness. You might also sometimes feel like a phony. When you believe in what you have been taught and become more competent, you become more confident. While providing therapy can be demanding, it is enormously gratifying. In this chapter, I share what some colleagues and I have experienced due to the nature of the work. I will digress at times to offer some practical tips.

Lack of validation may fuel self-doubt.

If you scored 95% on a test when you were a student, your performance was immediately confirmed. Others did not dispute it. You could compare scores with classmates and feel confident.

Now a client may grade you on the internet, not come back, or not pay you. They may even sue you. Most of the time, there is no concrete feedback. The progress you and your client are hoping for may take time. The limits you set on your client's acting-out behavior may sometimes lead to eventual improvement but result in an immediate negative response from the client.

The lack of validation can fuel self-doubt as you realize that the skills you gained as an excellent student don't always translate into being an effective therapist. Unlike simply studying, being an effective therapist requires you to apply what you've learned, develop broad social skills, and have insight into your client's dynamics and your own.

Beginners rely on their teachers' wisdom and their client's grace.

You can share your experiences with coworkers when you are part of a treatment team. However, many therapists work in isolation, which can be lonely.

Self-doubt and the characteristic uncertainty of therapy can affect your relationship with the client. You may feel vulnerable or intimidated.

Being a beginner worsens those effects. I looked over my shoulder the first time a client called me a doctor. I wanted to see who they were talking to. Indeed, I didn't think they could be talking to me.

As a beginning psychiatric resident working with clients who had much more life experience, I wondered how I could have the audacity to tell them anything. I had to remind myself that my authority came from the wisdom of my teachers and the literature I had studied. It helped that I had ready access to supervision when I had a question.

As a junior medical student, I had to wake patients early and draw blood. Patients at this teaching hospital allowed supervised medical students and residents to provide treatment. Often, these patients were older, weary, disadvantaged people suffering from the effects of multiple serious illnesses. Unfortunately, it takes practice to find a vein.

My lack of skill initially resulted in many sticks, and patients experienced needless pain. I learned a valuable lesson: Inexperience can hurt patients. I still feel indebted to these patients who allowed me to learn at their expense. That gift comes with an obligation to give the best care I can—a duty other therapists feel as well.

Decision-making can be daunting in a complex field with intrinsic uncertainties.

Part of your experience of doing therapy involves trying to become knowledgeable in a field exploding with information. It can be overwhelming. The complexity of things becomes more apparent. With that recognition comes a growing awareness of how it is impossible to know precisely how a client may respond.

For example, to prescribe the correct dose of a medication, I must ask myself a series of questions:

- What is the client's age?
- What is the client's total body water, in which the medication will be diluted?
- Does the medication like to be bound to fat cells? How much fat does the client have?
- How closely bound is the medication to the protein carrier? Will another medication the client is taking bump it off, making it more active in the blood?
- How will the client's sex affect their drug response?
- What enzyme systems are used in the liver to metabolize this drug? Is the client a slow or fast metabolizer in those systems?
- What medication is the client taking, and how is each metabolized?
- Do these other medications inhibit or increase the rate of metabolism of the drug I am prescribing?
- Has the client been allergic to a similar drug?

With these many factors, I cannot be sure whether a particular dose is best. If I have the luxury of starting low and slowly going up on dose while monitoring closely, I do. But sometimes, the severity of the illness won't allow me that luxury.

While some situations are more straightforward, I often must determine risk and benefit based on probabilities. It's unnerving to feel I am gambling with someone else's well-being.

Some things are more straightforward, but you often must become comfortable with uncertainty because it's part of the mystery characteristic of humanity.

Mistaken assumptions surprise therapists.

I discovered the hard way that I did not understand what it was like to be anxious. I quit drinking coffee for a month. Then I had a large cup. I had a full-fledged panic attack. There I was, a forty-year-old psychiatrist, beside myself with anxiety. I knew it was a panic attack, but it still felt unbearable. I felt like I was going to die or lose it.

This experience was the anxiety I had been hearing about for years. Up to then, I'd thought anxiety was a kind of heightened uneasiness that I felt before taking exams. Oh, no! That was not it at all! I will never quit drinking coffee again. There are so many clients I would have given a minor tranquilizer to had I known what this kind of anxiety is like.

When you have learned what you can but must make treatment decisions based on partial knowledge, you realize that you are making assumptions about what you don't know. It is natural to think other people's experiences are like your own. That's why I made incorrect assumptions about panic.

As you become more experienced, become more competent, and learn your strengths and weaknesses, you will enjoy what you do more and be more effective. But there will always be surprises.

Being proactive reduces the
likelihood of therapist burnout.

Many therapists are responding to a deep urge to help others when they choose to become therapists. When a therapist witnesses unavoidable suffering but can do little to alter the outcome, they suffer vicariously. They begin to comprehend, for example, how the mother in poverty suffers more from seeing her child go hungry than from the pain in her own stomach. Vicarious suffering, while intrinsic to therapy, can contribute to burnout.

Recognizing your limitations and planning around them can reduce the risk of burnout.

To offer a more down-to-earth example, don't schedule your difficult client first thing if you're not a morning person. If you feel like your brain and best judgment are giving out by late afternoon, don't schedule a difficult patient for that slot.

If you have a client who requires more time because of their complexity, consider scheduling a more extended session or seeing them before lunch. If you run over, it shortens lunch, but the delay for each successive appointment is not that significant.

Set limits on your client's discussion so you can make notes at the end of the session and consolidate what you just learned. If you tend to run over appointment times, consider using a timer or asking staff to ring you.

Your staff should feel you are approachable when they need to alert you to a crisis. On the other hand, you don't want them to think you are a pushover when they want to inject a client into your crowded schedule.

Setting limits on staff and clients helps you avoid being overextended. Let your clients know that they will benefit from you being refreshed and rested. That's how you can do your best to help them.

Saying no can be a means of letting the client know you believe in their competence to cope in a particular situation without you.

Work situations often don't allow for adequate breaks. So don't squander the breaks you do get by checking your cell or trying to multitask during them. Stop for a minute and just breathe. A therapist once told me that he had taken comfort in going to the bathroom because his day had been so hard. For just a moment, he could rejoice in feeling he knew exactly what he was doing.

Fear of being sued can add to your burnout, even if therapists are not sued as frequently as physicians. Lawyers will tell you that you are more likely to be sued if there are both bad feelings and a bad outcome. Some bad outcomes may be unavoidable. But when you demonstrate to your client and their family that you care about them and are trying your best, their bad feelings might be lessened.

You may not always have control over the outcome, but you can proactively create warm feelings. Knowing that you have adequate malpractice insurance and that your practice conforms to the usual practice in your community can be reassuring.

The client who sues you must prove that:

- You had a duty to them.
- You neglected your duty.
- There was some damage done.
- Your dereliction of duty directly caused that damage.

Keeping thorough documentation, staying current with developments in your field, and staying competent will reduce your risk of being successfully sued.

Being caught between your client and their physician can be stressful.

When your client's physician is not listening to your client and is possibly missing a diagnosis or prescribing the wrong treatment, it is stressful to feel some responsibility. Still, you may lack the power to effect a change.

There may be some things you can do to increase the chance that the physician will listen to you. But you will need your client's permission to discuss their case.

You might talk to the physician's office manager about the best time to speak with the doctor on the phone. Some doctors take time at lunch, while others save everything for the end of the day or a specific day of the week. Some days of the week might be horrendous. A doctor is more likely to feel imposed upon if they are asked to speak to someone when they have no time budgeted for it.

Doctors appreciate it when you present your case succinctly. But you also want to start by acknowledging the positive efforts the physician has already made. You hope to persuade them to agree with you without losing face.

Consider whether it would make sense to send the doctor a concise discussion of your concerns before your phone call so they have a chance to think about your points ahead of time. This is particularly appropriate if the case is complex and does not lend itself to a quick explanation. It also creates a document for your records.

In group practices, a specific nurse may be assigned to assist the doctor. I have found that I have more time to explain my case when I talk to the nurse. Nurses know the best time during the day to discuss messages with the doctor. The doctor may be more receptive to your message when it comes from the nurse, who has an everyday working relationship with them and best knows how to couch different ideas.

Doctors are often impressed with a therapist's concern and the efforts they've made to collaborate in the treatment. You will sometimes be surprised at the difference between what the doctor said and what the client heard. Document your efforts and what was discussed in your progress notes.

Suicidal clients heighten a therapist's feelings of responsibility and command their best judgment and careful attention to detail.

I heard a version of a story about Alabama football coach Bear Bryant. Bear rarely lost games. A commentator asked him why he lost a recent game. Coach replied that his team did not lose the game. The officials had called time before his team could win.

When I work with suicidal clients, I fear that they will call time before I have had a chance to help them win. It is hard to know with any certainty how much time there is left in the game. That's scary.

The stakes are so high. When it comes to treatment, the consequences of making a mistake in judgment are immeasurable. Learn as much as you can from multiple sources about assessing suicidal risk and the risk of violence.

Therapists muster courage, self-confidence, and some detachment to take on risks.

As a student, I worked as a surgical technician for some summers. I came to appreciate what a surgeon goes through when they make that first cut and open the abdomen. There could be surprises. Human anatomy varies. Patients' heart-lung capacities vary. Some patients bleed more. A surgeon must believe they can do what they need to and then close the abdomen with the patient still alive.

I like to call that belief "necessary narcissism." Perhaps the word *narcissism* is a little harsh and inaccurate. Still, I use it to emphasize that a bit of grandiosity and a sense of omnipotence can be helpful and even necessary. It allows the surgeon to be somewhat detached from their emotions about the potential consequences of what they are doing. Those feelings during surgery would be distracting.

It is like whistling in the dark to feel less vulnerable about being alone in the dark. If surgeons weren't courageous enough to take those risks, patients could not benefit. You show a similar courage when you take up the mantle of clinical responsibility.

Sometimes, praise makes therapists feel like imposters.

Eventually, with hard work, you can base your confidence in your abilities on your knowledge and competence. But until you get there, there may be times when you feel like an imposter.

Arlin Cuncic with Verywellmind has written an interesting article about imposter syndrome: "Is Imposter Syndrome Holding You Back from Living Your Best Life?" Here is the link: https://www.verywellmind.com/imposter-syndrome-and-social-anxiety-disorder-4156469 (Cuncic 2024).

According to Cuncic, if you aren't perfect, don't know everything about the subject, need help, or aren't superbly accomplished, you may feel like an imposter and fear being exposed.

You also read Martin Huecker et al.'s article "Imposter Phenomenon" at https://www.ncbi.nlm.nih.gov/books/NBK585058/ for additional information.

My pathology professor at the Medical College of Georgia, Dr. Luther Otkin, told medical students that, contrary to popular belief, doctors don't think they are God. He said they believe they are disciples of medicine. As I mentioned earlier, my faith in the people who taught me and what they taught me helped me think that what I was doing would work. It wasn't so much that I believed in myself, but rather that I believed in the practice of medicine itself.

Angry clients can make
therapists feel vulnerable.

We all make mistakes. The wrong medication is chosen. Our clients will be justifiably mad at us. We may become defensive, and our expressions will give us away.

Clients may be upset with you for being late, charging them too much, making them pay for missed sessions, or not being able to see them sooner. You may feel like running away or taking a nap. You model how to handle anger when you handle theirs. Show genuine curiosity about why they are angry with you. Work with them to puzzle about it. Sometimes, it is apparent. You'll need to apologize, or maybe not. Some clients will forgive you, and others will hold a grudge. All is grist for the therapy mill.

Sometimes, clients are mad at someone else. The world is unfair, and they may have been mistreated, abused, etc. Validate them. You may want to match their tone and gradually de-escalate it. Avoid them becoming enraged and dangerous. Perhaps you don't get what they are trying to tell you. Take a neutral stance as you encourage them to be curious about it.

It is natural to want your clients to like you. Of course, you don't want them to be mad at you or dissatisfied. This natural tendency makes you want to placate the client or become defensive. But sometimes, you must wear a black hat and set limits on a client's behaviors.

Even if a client is not mad at you, you may feel uncomfortable in the presence of a client who is mad about something else. Their anger may be justified or not. Being in the presence of an angry client may trigger memories of a past exposure to people who were out of control.

Maybe you have not had those experiences and are not used to being around tension and conflict. It may take practice to become more comfortable. Your job is to help clients put their feelings into words and not into behavior or acting out.

Dependent and narcissistic clients produce heroic feelings in therapists.

You are not the only one who needs to believe in you. Your clients also need to believe in you. They don't want to think there are gaps in your abilities. For example, no one has ever asked me if I graduated in the bottom half of my medical class, even though there is a fifty-fifty chance that any doctor has.

The client's tendency to ascribe authority to you, whether deserved or not, can feel reinforcing and emotionally reassuring in the face of your daunting task. It's so tempting to fall into the role of a hero!

My family has helped dispel any illusions I might have of being a hero. When I open the door to my home, I enter a world where I am the husband who forgot to pick up bread and has not mastered how to load the dishwasher properly.

When you feel that a client has idealized you, ask yourself if this client is dependent and expects you to do the work. Similarly, narcissistic clients will see you as an extension of themselves. So they see you as flawless too.

Stigma, geographical separation, and confidentiality requirements can isolate therapists.

It is crucial to have connections with colleagues because confidentiality significantly limits what you can say to your family about your work. Regularly meeting with work colleagues or a supervisor can help you feel less isolated. As a therapist, you are part of your tool kit. Being in therapy yourself can help you know yourself better and sharpen that tool.

If you encounter a client in public, do not acknowledge that you know them unless they choose to recognize you. That preserves their privacy and avoids subjecting them to stigma.

When I set up my first private practice in a small, rural town, I discovered that townspeople went to my colleague in a village thirty miles away. Her townspeople traveled to my town to see me. People did not want to be seen coming into our offices.

I raised sheep on my twelve-acre farm a few miles from town. I moved my office to the first floor of my old farmhouse, which was built into the bank of a hill. People from my village were willing to come and see me. Scheduling people could be tricky because they did not want to face someone they knew.

There is quiet satisfaction associated with doing effective therapy.

Being a therapist may be challenging, but it is worthwhile. Seeing your clients make better decisions, become better partners or parents, and avoid making the same mistakes again is gratifying. When you help clients put the puzzle pieces together, you share in their excitement at the discovery. Imagine knowing you helped a young person reach their potential and changed the direction of their life. Feeling valued by your clients is also rewarding.

Your clients will teach you much about life. The relationships you have with them will enrich it.

So many therapists are wonderful people, and *you* get to work with them. The camaraderie and sense of working on a shared mission can be inspiring and fun. There is pride in belonging to the profession. The tools available to therapists are continually improving. Using those new tools to benefit a client is exhilarating.

In this chapter: We took a glimpse into therapists' feelings.

In the next chapter: We will examine the client's feelings about therapy and the prospect of change. You will read about clients who don't want to be aware of their dynamics, do not see their behavior as maladaptive, lack hope of changing, or resent being told what to do.

Chapter 15

Discerning Clients' Resistance to Treatment

Multiple elements go into a client's resistance to change, including major mental illness, physical factors, medication effects, protective denial, lack of skills and knowledge, immaturity, passive-aggressiveness, and oppositional tendencies.

Multiple forces go into a client's resistance to change.

Many of your clients might belong to the "worried well" and have skills and maturity. They are willing to look at themselves. These attributes make therapy easier. But as excited as clients are about changing, some things may stand in their way.

Imagine you are using your hand to prop up a pencil against a clipboard that is held at a sixty-degree angle. Your hand is just beneath the pencil, and the force of gravity holds the pencil against it. The force you exert upward against the pencil keeps it from sliding downward. Cohesive forces in the pencil keep it from falling apart. Air flows by the pencil. The sum of the forces on it is equal, causing it to stay put. It is stuck. The pencil appears to be inactive, yet many forces are at work. If we ascribe a motive to the pencil, we might say it is a lazy pencil that does not want to move. We might say that the forces on it conflict with one another.

The pencil moves when you remove one of those forces by taking your hand away. It is no longer resistant to change.

Clients are aware of some behavioral determinants, but not others.

Multiple forces also affect people's resistance to change. We describe behavior as "multi-determined." Clients are unaware of some of these behavioral determinants.

Current research shows that our brains have billions of nerve cells. So, much activity goes on at the same time. We can't be aware of all the multiple psychological processes in our brains, both waking and sleeping, that affect our behavior.

We cannot be sure what someone is thinking or why they feel what they do. This uncertainty is part of our challenge in trying to understand and help others.

The unconscious is not located in a specific part of the brain. The term refers to that part of the mind that is not accessible. Over the years, people have developed mental constructs to understand what is happening in the unconscious. We call these constructs "psychodynamics," or "dynamics" for short. We try to understand the client's dynamics by examining how one thought leads to another. When they repeat behaviors, we look for themes in the patterns. We examine how their view of us recreates past conflictual relationships.

Clients defend against recognizing their dynamics.

Understanding the unconscious dynamics allows us to help the client become aware of them, make better choices, and avoid repeating maladaptive behaviors. Removing resistance is like taking your hand away from the pencil and freeing it up to move. Freed from the effort needed to remain unaware, they develop a more accurate understanding of themselves. And that leads to change.

The process of becoming aware of dynamics can make a client anxious. Developing an excellent client-therapist relationship is essential because the client needs to feel safe and have a caring, competent, and careful therapist they can talk freely to. Ideally, you will have helped the client develop techniques to deal with the anxiety and contain the generated affect.

"The process of psychotherapy is to strengthen the ego to be able to hear what one does not want to hear—the worst thing one could hear—what one's defenses were erected to prevent" (Dill 2022).

Clients may feel they are paying a lot to see you and want to get into the heavy stuff right away. They may expect a quick fix. Let them know that you will work with them to develop the skills they need to cope with the resultant anxiety and difficult emotions. Explain the importance of developing skills and a sense of safety before diving into the more challenging material.

Clients use different defense mechanisms to avoid the anxiety that comes with becoming aware. These defenses include some combination of denial, projection, displacement, regression, rationalization, reaction formation, repression, or sublimation.

Ryan Baily and Jose Pico discuss these and other defense mechanisms in StatPearls at https://www.ncbi.nlm.nih.gov/books/NBK559106/ (Bailey and Pico 2025).

Resistance is not just a roadblock. It's also the stuff of therapy and not just the roadblocks. If you have ever played the game Battleship, you know that if you accidentally set off a mine planted by your opponent, you also discover where their battleship is. You know they put their mines near their battleships to protect them. Similarly, when you encounter your client's resistance, you know that something there is important.

Let's look at how clients may resist treatment. They may have varying degrees of awareness of their resistance.

Reluctance to change may not be because of psychological resistance.

If your client does not understand what you are saying or misunderstands you, they may have a subtle hearing deficit. Hearing impairment is not always related to age. Hunters, service members, and rock concert fans are at risk. Clients may fill in the gap with assumptions based on what they expect you to say. Sometimes, they may look a little paranoid. Do you often have to repeat what you say?

English may be the client's second language. When I am in another country and don't quite understand what a salesclerk is saying, I smile and act like what I missed was not essential. Clients may also misread your behavior and manners.

When a client looks unmotivated, they may have a physical illness that makes them tired. Everything, including therapy, is more challenging when fatigued. Consider whether they may benefit from a workup for long-term COVID-19, anemia, hypothyroidism, diabetes, hepatitis, sleep apnea, mononucleosis, heart disease, poor nutrition, or low testosterone.

Marijuana can cause amotivational syndrome. Anergia (extreme persistent fatigue) can be a symptom of clinical depression and several other diseases. Apathy can be a symptom of several diseases, including neurological disease.

Robert van Reekum et al. have written an excellent article on apathy titled "Apathy: Why Care?" (Reekum 2005). Here is the link: https://psychiatryonline.org/doi/full/10.1176/jnp.17.1.7.

Sometimes, clients feel that if they talk, they risk being rejected by their family. Families may not approve of therapy or medications that affect the brain. They may feel threatened, knowing that secrets about abuse, addiction, infidelity, sexual abuse, or mental illness may come out. Family members may also believe that a client who needs therapy lacks faith in God.

Some people lack opportunities that would lead to a sense of personal agency. It seems life will not work out for them no matter what they do. Because they're in pain, these clients may try therapy anyway. You may be the first person to believe in them, see their worth, or want to hear what they have to say. They may continue therapy, but it may be more because they like you than because they think they will succeed. They don't want to let you down because it seems to matter to you how well they do.

Some people are reluctant to do therapy due to realistic, common-sense reasons. You may not know that the things they need to change are monumental and personally costly to change. If that client makes a change, they may be going against their family or culture. In another example, a woman may not want to realize her spouse is unfaithful because that would mean having to leave him and become a single parent.

Too little or too much medication hinders therapy.

If a client is too nervous, they may not do psychotherapy. Conversely, overmedicated clients may lack the motivation to do psychotherapy.

Some clients don't recognize their maladaptive behaviors.

A client may see smoking or doing drugs as part of who they are and not a problem. They see the behaviors as ego-syntonic. Something that is ego-syntonic is thought to be consistent with the client's fundamental view of themselves and their beliefs.

Clients may feel that your focus on change implies that they are not good enough as they are. In reality, you are showing them that you accept them as a person, encourage their self-acceptance, and help them change maladaptive ways of thinking and behaving. You want them to see those maladaptive parts of themselves as ego-dystonic, or not consistent with their identity. Your compassion shows them that you accept them as they are. For example, you accept the smoker but not the behavior of smoking.

Your client's values may be different from yours, and your client may not have a concept of the value of therapy. Instead of being psychologically minded, maybe they have a superficial view of life. Because they see things concretely, they aren't aware of the psychological process. They don't consider personal growth an essential value. Clarifying these clients' goals for treatment may help you see how and where to begin.

Different situations require different approaches to denial.

When a client sees maladaptive behaviors as part of themselves, this is just one form of denial. Denial is an unwillingness to accept reality and acknowledge what others can see as fact. It's a defense mechanism against anxiety, but it also leads to resistance to change. If a client can't conceptualize a problem as a problem, they don't see it and can't address it.

Their brain may have repressed something by pushing the anxiety-producing thought into their unconscious. The memory is not available to let them put a piece in the puzzle.

Imagine a half-ton pickup truck. How much manure can it haul? The answer is an infinity of manure, but only an average of three thousand pounds at a time. If you pile too much manure on it, it will break down from the load.

Sometimes, a person feels so bad about themselves, their life, and what they have done or not done that they already have three thousand pounds of emotional manure on their pickup truck. You may need to help them remove some of the more reachable emotional manure and reinforce the pickup truck before you consider breaking through their denial. Prematurely breaking through their denial is like reminding a tightrope walker how high up they are.

When I was working in a senior intensive outpatient program, I met a woman who, as a child, had to wear worn-out, hand-me-down clothes to school. Her lifelong sense of shame manifested as an inability to protect herself from being used by others. When she entered treatment, confrontation was not part of her treatment.

Instead, she took part in group therapy several times weekly with other clients from her community. She discovered similarities with other group members and made strong connections. She witnessed them being cared about and accepted for who they were. In time, she came to feel accepted for herself. It was only then that her denial broke. Then she could see how shame had compromised her ability to set limits on others. Being accepted by others opened the way for her to accept the orphaned parts of herself.

On the other hand, my experiences in inpatient addiction treatment emphasized the need to break through denial more quickly because the denied behaviors were dangerous. These clients were in a supervised, safe setting with supportive staff, and intensive treatment was readily available. Staff carefully monitored the treatment effects. Clients were encouraged to see the big picture, remember their strengths, and be aware of their support network as they examined the consequences of their behaviors.

Clients may not have developed the personal skill set to do therapy or initially see its value.

Ideally, children learn frustration tolerance by having to tolerate incrementally more difficult, age-appropriate frustration. If their parents do not provide them with opportunities to develop this tolerance, they may lack ego strength. People with ego strength can tolerate frustration, compromise, reflect on themselves, and see the big picture. These are the very skills clients need to do therapy successfully.

Clients who have a dim awareness of their skills gaps prefer to maintain the status quo and avoid taking on responsibilities they cannot manage. Instead, they expect others to change. Beneath their voiced entitlement is an unrecognized feeling of inadequacy. By providing emotional support and using parent-like therapy techniques, you could gradually empower them by patiently helping them develop the ego strength they need to do the work in small steps.

Clients lacking self-reliance may be reluctant to accept responsibility for themselves.

Some people have a stronger aggressive drive than others. They have agency, take ownership of their therapy, and actively participate in the process. Other people are more passive and feel they are not the hero of their life story. They don't want to be the alpha dog and prefer being taken care of. They want someone else to be responsible. Their situation growing up may not have supported their incremental growth toward self-reliance.

If you are feeling unusually maternal, ask yourself if the client is encouraging you to take care of them and do the work of therapy. They may think that doing the work themselves will risk you abandoning them, as they will no longer need you.

Passive-aggressive clients express their aggression by withholding progress.

When people are not comfortable expressing their aggression directly, they may express it passively by withholding, like a two-year-old child who withholds pooping in the toilet during toilet training. If a client consistently comes late, forgets their credit card, and requires you to pull teeth to get them to talk, they may be passive-aggressive. They may show subtle contempt by not bothering to bathe or change clothes. (Some depressed clients find activities of daily living to take too much effort. So make sure your client is not depressed.)

Do you feel irritated? Do they seem to get some pleasure from defeating you, the person they see as their opponent in the tug-of-war? Hearing them talk about how their boss or spouse is frustrated with them may make it clear that understanding the passive-aggressive behavior is central to the therapy.

Set limits on your passive-aggressive client so they can't externalize their conflict by putting their feelings into behavior. When they can't act out, they will internalize the conflict and make progress. When I worked in a prison setting, I noticed how depressed prisoners became when the acting out was limited and they realized their internal conflicts.

Clients become defensive if they believe you are telling them what to do or think.

Even when you listen carefully, ask open-ended questions, and pose your statements as ideas to consider, the client may feel you are telling them what to do. They resent it. Clients who had controlling parents may believe that you also think you know best and that you want to impose your opinion on them.

Victims of prejudice may expect you to act superior and discount their views. Their reflex opposition may reflect growing self-worth.

To avoid looking pretentious and authoritarian, I dress plainly in clothes that might have come off the rack at Walmart. My standard garb is an old, gray button-up sweater reminiscent of Mr. Rogers. It makes me look kind and nonthreatening. I want my clients to think it is going to be a "wonderful day in the neighborhood" and not a day at the office with a competitive male coworker or sexually abusive boss. I operate from a one-down position to be approachable and encourage emotional comfort.

In other settings, I might wear a suit because upscale clients would consider me unprofessional if I dressed otherwise and discount what I said.

I want my clients to feel safe. I speak softly, move slowly, and sit comfortably back in my chair. My responses to their comments are not rapid and may include a pause that shows I am carefully considering what they just said. I recognize that I might seem threatening, so my verbal and nonverbal behaviors anticipate that.

Oppositional behavior may have several explanations.

Occasionally, a client will loudly object to everything you say, including your recommendations. If they have a history of this exact behavior over time, consider whether they have oppositional defiant disorder (ODD). Clients with ODD tend to be grumpy, argumentative, and even spiteful at times.

Sometimes, clients who are manic can't listen and are very sure of their own opinions.

Some people with schizophrenia are negativistic, and that negativism can look superficially like ODD.

While autistic clients vary widely, some have pathological demand avoidance, which results in them perceiving requests as a threat to their autonomy. Occasionally, autistic clients think your requests are illogical and should not be followed.

Don't equate opposition or rigidity with invulnerability. Some rigid clients are fragile.

There is a group of people who come across as very rigid. Because they are so very inflexible, you may at first think they are solid. In fact, behind their rigid defenses, they are fragile. You need to treat them gently and work hard to avoid saying anything that could feel like a slight. They are easily narcissistically wounded. They are like peanut brittle. Brittle things are both rigid and fragile. They break easily.

Involuntary clients may have trouble changing due to serious mental illness.

Your voluntary outpatient client has made some effort to get up, dress, travel to your office, set aside time, and prepare to pay you. These behaviors suggest motivation to change and a desire for something to be different.

On the other hand, involuntary clients may lack the motivation and even partial insight that outpatient clients have. Some involuntary clients are, by definition, a potential danger to themselves or others. They may be psychotic, intoxicated, manic, profoundly depressed, suicidal, or unbearably anxious. Hopefully, medical interventions, medications, close observation, and support will make them more amenable to therapy at some point.

A discussion of serious mental illness (SMI) and inpatient treatment is beyond this book's scope. Your first exposure to severe mental illness can be overwhelming. Harry Stack Sullivan said, "We are all more simply human than otherwise."

That is a good thing to remember as you see clients who are on the wrong side of the locked door.

In this chapter: I proposed that clients, like the lazy pencil, may have multiple opposing forces that hold them in place. I suggested that you look for language and hearing problems, physical illness, apathy, rational fear of unwanted consequences, and pathological demand avoidance as plausible explanations for their resistance. I noted that anxiety, hopelessness, rigidity, and unawareness of their behavior's maladaptive quality may contribute to their resistance.

In the next chapter: We focus on how the client's and therapist's unconscious thoughts and feelings contribute to resistance to changing the client's compulsive, repetitive behaviors.

Chapter 16

The Interplay of Transference and Countertransference

Therapists use their understanding of transference, countertransference, and client dynamics to identify the sources of the client's compulsive, repetitive behaviors.

Underneath the happenings in therapy is an unconscious process. It may differ from the superficial content.

In the interaction between you and the client, the content is apparent, but the process is not always obvious. This reminds me of a story about a mother and her schizophrenic son who were eating in the hospital cafeteria. Staff overheard the mother telling her son how important it was for him to become mature and independent. Her words surprised the staff because she was cutting up his meat for him as she spoke. The content of her speech contradicted her actions, leaving the son with a mixed message.

The therapist examines the unconscious sources of resistance.

Transference and countertransference are part of the process of psychotherapy. Ralph Greenson states, "Transference refers to all the feelings the client is experiencing toward the therapist, which are displaced from figures in the past." He adds that "some feelings are appropriate and realistic based on the actual behavior of the therapist."

He goes on to explain, "Countertransference is based on the unconscious conflicts in the therapist's past which make him react to the client as though the client was a significant figure in the therapist's past" (Greenson, pp 1399–1415, 1959).

The word *counter* is misleading. The countertransference is not against the client's transference.

To understand the client's resistance to developing a more rational ego, the therapist explores the transference and the countertransference.

Psychoanalytic technique is designed to elucidate the transference and use that to understand the nature of the client's resistance to developing a more rational ego. (Very simply put, in theory, the ego is that part of the personality that is aware of the self and tries to make realistic compromises between wishes and learned rules of behavior.)

While a nonanalytic therapist would not necessarily focus on this, understanding how transference, resistance, and countertransference work helps them understand the client.

Identifying the significant figures in a client's past and their emotional response to them helps you understand what the client is reliving in the present. The repetition compulsion is the tendency to recreate and repeat conflictual situations to relive rather than remember the original one.

The positive transference works toward therapeutic progress. The negative transference, with its anger, mistrust, and hostility, hinders it. For example, in a negative transference, the client may see you as judgmental, like earlier significant figures, and feel reluctant to trigger your critical judgment by disclosing shortcomings.

I encourage you to read Dr. Greenson's article to get a more precise, less simplified discussion of transference and countertransference. You might also want to read Dr. J. D. Gill's refreshingly lucid explanations in her book *Doing Psychotherapy: A Primer*.

I want to look broadly at reactions or assumptions that you and a client can make about each other based not only on past figures but also on different experiences and cultural influences. Technically, that is not transference or countertransference. These reactions may be a mixture that includes or is shaped by transference/countertransference. Behavior is multi-determined. So, multiple influences, both conscious and unconscious, shape behavior.

**Bret's and Myrtle's cases
illustrate how transference and
countertransference operate in therapy.**

I entered my waiting room to hear the loud voice of my new client, Bret, who was chatting up my secretary. I noticed her taking in how tightly his tailored shirt and khaki slacks accentuated his build. He was dropping the names of prominent townspeople who had gone with him to see his team play in the national football championship. He took his eyes off my secretary long enough to look up and say, "Hi, Doc." (I hate being called "Doc" almost as much as the character Doc Martin did on TV. It feels demeaning.) I could feel the muscles in my jaw tighten a bit, but I was determined to remain courteous anyway.

As he entered my office, Bret immediately remarked on the size of my desk. It was a large piece of wood that I'd had a local carpenter finish and lacquer. It rested on two short filing cabinets. Bret seemed put off by my lack of an executive-style desk. I detected a slight grimace when he had to sit down in one of my rocking chairs. He was sizing up the competition and trying to assess my status.

I was a loser.

Bret explained he was a successful business executive who, at fifty-five, had a young wife he was trying to keep happy. It was her idea that he go to therapy. She had told him he wasn't himself, as if he was losing a step.

As I asked about symptoms, I was careful to couch my language in noncritical words, even though I'd already felt put off by Bret's behavior. Nonetheless, he was defensive and seemed to think he needed to compete with me. He noted my college diploma and reminded me that his school had defeated mine in an important basketball game. Eventually, he seemed to realize that I was not a threat and had been pointing out some of his strengths.

Over time, it became more apparent that Bret had a very critical father who expected success from his son, whom he saw as an extension of himself. Bret could never please him. And now, as he got older, he was having problems pleasing his wife. His transference feelings about me involved seeing me as a critical authority figure who was an opponent he would have to compete against.

My countertransference involved my feelings about the jocks in my high school who had picked on me, an eighth-grade student council nerd who was unsuccessfully trying to keep them from smoking in the school bathroom. In my gut, I felt Bret was subtly going to bully me for not being an athlete. Knowing I was most certainly a nerd and not a jock put my masculinity in question and played into my adolescent issues with self-worth.

So, Bret had been bullied by his father, and jocks had bullied me. In time, Bret became more accepting of himself, understood how his father's insecurities affected their relationship, felt less compelled to always be a winner, and realized that his wife loved him for who he was. As I got to know him better, I found myself more sympathetic to his vulnerability and able to be genuinely accepting of him.

The conscious process was talking about solving Bret's problem of not feeling like himself, but the unconscious process involved the transference/countertransference issues around bullying and self-acceptance.

You'll be glad to know that I got over my issue with jocks. My wife is a jock who played college basketball and coached high school basketball. I won't let her smoke in the bathroom.

Like Bert, Myrtle was defensive

Another transference and countertransference occurred when I saw Myrtle, a forty-five-year-old single woman who worked for our local veterinarian. She had unkempt hair and wore drab, loose-fitting scrubs from work. Her appearance seemed to be saying, "Not interested."

She told me she got along better with animals than people and was having problems with her coworkers, whom she described as sneaky, two-faced bitches. She said she felt like there were two kinds of people: bad people and bad people pretending to be good.

It did not take long for me to see that Myrtle suspected I was the latter. After all, she was paying me to be nice. It was not so much that she was paranoid (thinking people were out to get her) as it was that she saw people as simply bad and uncaring.

Eventually, she could tell me that her father had abused her when she was an early adolescent and that her mother hadn't believed her. Her transference to me was to suspect that I would eventually abuse her and discount what she told me.

My countertransference was feeling irritated, as I had with a girlfriend who questioned the intent behind everything I did.

If I did something nice for her, she thought I wanted something from her or had ulterior motives.

> Deirdre's, Selma's, and Harriet's cases
> illustrate how clients unconsciously
> repeat behaviors to master them.

When someone sees a spotted four-legged animal coming at them quickly from three hundred yards away, they sort through profiles of animals—four-legged animals, fast-moving animals, and spotted animals—to decide if it is a leopard. Then they become terrified and run. Their mind assumes things based on experience and reading, and they react accordingly. They have benefited from what they learned in the past.

When a small child uses trial and error to learn how to pour milk, they repeat their behavior and eventually learn from the repetitions to pour milk without spilling it.

In both instances—seeing the leopard and pouring the milk— the person is consciously trying to apply what they learned in the past to deal with the present task. Sometimes, there are unconscious processes outside awareness that are factors in that behavior.

Sometimes, people unwittingly feel compelled to repeat their behavior to master an unconscious conflict. Each time they repeat the behavior, they try to benefit from what they learned the previous time.

The repetition compulsion is a friend to the investigating therapist, but not to the client's progress. In the transference, the client recreates the most recent compulsive repetition of the earlier conflictual relationship. The therapist then uses the most recent example of the behavior to look back in time for analogous situations—earlier repetitions. The client may show similar behaviors toward other people and in different situations.

Take Deirdre, for example. Faultlessly dressed and with artful makeup, my thirtyish client told me she regularly worked out, tried to stay fit, and was sexually available to her boyfriend. Despite this, her boyfriend was constantly distant and self-absorbed. She wondered whether she had been attentive enough to his needs, yet she also felt he should reciprocate her affection.

Deirdre's girlfriends had warned her that he was just like her last boyfriend, whom they described as creepy and cold. They had pushed another guy on her, but she said he was just too sweet, and she didn't feel any spark of attraction.

Her mom and dad had divorced after her mom had an affair, claiming she had finally found a man who could love her. Her dad had spent more time in the garage than with his family and seemed to care more about his Mustang than them. To no avail, Deirdre had taken an automotive class in high school, hoping they could work on the car together.

Deirdre was trying to master the unconscious conflict of getting someone unloving and distant to love her. She sought distant men to recreate the situation and master it. But she was only vaguely aware of this. The clue was that nice guys did not excite her. In the transference, she discounted any positive thing I said because I was a nice guy and not distant. She did not want acceptance from me. Deirdre wanted it from someone aloof and indifferent.

Some of the mixed feelings clients have toward therapists and the assumptions they make about them come from popular culture.

Therapists are depicted as benign but lacking common sense, sociopathic, powerful mind readers, wise but different, boundary violators, greedy, clueless, arrogant, and amazingly insightful about others but deeply flawed themselves.

In your first meeting with a client, you will orient the client to what therapy is and explain your standard procedures. That may reassure them that you don't fit into one of those stereotypes. Don't give in to the temptation to explain more about yourself than you need to. It may feel like you are rudely withholding part of yourself. But you are declining to show your hand for a therapeutic reason. The more concrete things the client knows about you, the more artifacts you introduce into the transference. For example, if they know you have a child, they can't imagine that you are unable to have children.

They may already have information about you, especially if you live in a small town or if they found you through a friend or the internet. You may not avoid them seeing your wedding ring, but think twice about putting family pictures on your desk or stickers on your car.

Besides looking for a wedding ring, clients may look at what you are wearing to see if how you dress is signaling sexual interest. So, avoid wearing anything that could be perceived as sexual.

Clients have preconceived notions about therapists based on what others have told them.

Clients may have culturally based prejudices against you because of sex, gender, sexual orientation, race, relationship status, ethnicity, religion, age, appearance, and other characteristics.

When I worked at the US Public Health Service Hospital in Baltimore, my boss required us to wear our uniforms once a week. I had seen Selma, the wife of a retired army sergeant, for several Tuesdays. She had remarked about how easy it was to talk to me.

Then Selma came on a Wednesday and saw me wearing an officer's uniform. All her feelings about officers, which had grown out of listening to her husband talk about officers for years, surfaced. Her husband had portrayed officers as snobbish know-it-alls who were clueless about how things should be run yet always found fault in the recruits. Selma suspected that I looked down on her after hearing her admit to her shortcomings. She thought I had cynically feigned my acceptance of her. She felt I had somehow tricked her into talking to an officer. Our sessions were never the same after that.

Clients may unconsciously count on you to be invulnerable, as they counted on their parents as children.

There will be times over your career when you miss work because of illness, accidents, family illness, or a death in the family. Clients may be surprised. They may be realistically concerned and show compassion and thoughtfulness to you and your family. Let them know you are thankful.

Here is an example of how you can learn something from your client's reactions.

Getting over an awful cold, I came to work one day feeling worn out, coughing, and frequently blowing my nose.

My appointment was with Harriet, a young woman who often came late to sessions and frequently wore something she had worn the day before and had just thrown on as she ran out the door. Scatterbrained, Harriet usually fumbled through sessions like she fumbled through life, seemingly without direction. But on this day, she was organized and goal-directed, putting together the things we had discussed in previous sessions and talking about her optimism. I wondered why there had been such a change.

Harriet had a mom who struggled with chronic depression and had difficulty being a mother. Harriet loved her mom and wished her mother could get it together to mother her better. Harriet saw I was having difficulty and had been trying to act in a way that made me feel better so I could better mother her.

My client's caring behavior was multi-determined. It reflected her human kindness, but her behavior also gave me insight into the mother-daughter relationship and her strong wish for a functional mother.

The first clue you might get about the transference is how you feel about the client. So, ask yourself, "What do I feel about the client?"

In this chapter: I defined and illustrated transference and countertransference, but they are not the only things going on in therapy.

In the next chapter: We begin a three-chapter exploration of the feelings the client and the therapist have about each other. Culture, situations, and client types all affect client-therapist interaction. I give two examples of the effect of culture. Aspects of culture may encourage a client to feel like a kid in the principal's office or like a customer.

Chapter 17

The Role of Cultural Stereotyping in Client-Therapist Interaction

The missing ingredient needed to figure out the client who stumps you could be the influence of culture.

Marginalized people show tremendous courage.

I work with people of diverse cultures, countries of origin, genders, races, sexual orientations, sexual preferences, and languages. At those times, I worry that I will put my foot in my mouth because I lack understanding and can engage in unthinking cultural stereotyping. My first thought might be to avoid talking about the differences and hope their problem relates to something else. However, when I acknowledge that I am aware that they belong to a marginalized group and ask if they have concerns related to that, I am letting them know that it is okay to talk about those concerns.

I am not surprised when they wait to see if I accept them because I see them in my heart as truly equal. They may suspect that, underneath, I believe I am better and am graciously deeming them acceptable from my position of superiority.

In today's political atmosphere, clients are looking for clues about you and your beliefs to gauge how safe it is to talk to you. They may have already been betrayed as they've tried to find their way through the assortment of therapists who pose as open-minded and well-intended but reject a marginalized client when the client discloses too much. Unfortunately, this guessing game has become necessary. But it delays treatment.

Clients reasonably expect that you are not only accepting but also have some knowledge and understanding of their group. When your client is aware of your knowledge, it helps them be more comfortable talking.

Creating an environment of emotional and physical safety is important for everyone, but even more so for marginalized people, who may have felt vulnerable in ways unknown to you. If you can, provide a quiet setting, comfortable chairs, warm furnishings, and adequate uninterrupted session time to talk. It can help if your client can sense sincere concern in your thorough attention to detail and calm in your tone of voice and lack of hurriedness. These elements can foster openness and a feeling of being considered and heard.

My diverse clients have graciously added to my knowledge. I have learned that each person and situation is complex and unique. This makes it hard to generalize about dynamics. But the one generalization I can confidently make is that marginalized people show a tremendous amount of courage in the face of hardship. This topic warrants more discussion than this book can provide. Instead, I offer some helpful resources in the appendix.

For some clients, seeing a therapist is like being sent to the principal's office.

As little kids, we tried new things we had never done before. We made mistakes. Lacking the impulse control or patience to wait for dinner, we snuck a cookie. As we continually did things wrong, it was easy to feel like we were bad for giving in to temptations. As adults, we remember getting caught and feeling bad about ourselves.

When I worked at a geriatric intensive outpatient program, clients came to my office for their regular visits. Some seemed to feel like they had been called into the principal's office. That little kid's feeling about being caught doing something wrong limited what they would tell me. They would insist that everything was just fine. Later, they would tell staff that their medication had side effects. They didn't feel comfortable with me until they'd had many visits and heard other clients say I was okay.

It helped that it wasn't me but their family doctor who prescribed medication. The client felt they could avoid the risk of getting sick from psychiatric medication I'd prescribed. They did not want the stigma of taking medication prescribed by a psychiatrist.

Emphasize to your clients the importance of reporting any health issues they experience, so you can help them prevent those issues from worsening.

Part of the clients' reluctance to see me in the communities where I have practiced has come from my being an outsider who seemed to peddle an invisible product.

It is easy for some clients to see themselves as your customer.

In our consumer-oriented society, several circumstances make it seem logical to clients that seeing a therapist is just one more shopping transaction. For example, we are now labeled as "providers." The first thing that comes up when clients present themselves to the office manager is payment for services. Clients may feel it is only natural for the provider, not the customer, to do the work. The customer paradigm encourages a sense of entitlement to a fast, straightforward solution.

Clients may believe that the provider picking out the right pill for them does not differ from a store clerk helping the shopper pick the right pair of shoes. It is challenging to explain the collaborative nature of therapy to clients who see themselves as consumers.

In this chapter: I hinted at how cultural influences might explain client behavior.

In the next chapter: I note some situations that lead to client-therapist interactions.

Chapter 18
Events That Happen During Therapy Shape Client-Therapist Interaction

Sometimes, the therapist creates a situation by making a mistake or taking a vacation. Other events come about when the client has a loss, becomes suicidal, or must be involuntarily admitted to the hospital.

Clarissa's case shows the importance of admitting mistakes.

It is not uncommon for clients to ask legitimate questions about your qualifications and training. You may also have to field intrusive questions about your personal life, religious beliefs, political affiliations, and past. Their questioning provides an immediate chance to explain how your client's knowledge of you limits the development of transference. Inquiring why they have asked a particular question may give a clue to their dynamics.

While you may sometimes withhold information about yourself for therapeutic reasons, clients rightly expect you to be honest. That means that when you make a mistake, you explain and apologize.

Clarissa was a graduate student in her mid-twenties who observed me treating her like she was much younger. She was exactly right. My frequent explanations would have been appropriate only if she had been one of the many eighteen-year-olds I was accustomed to treating. After admitting she was right to call me on it, I pledged to avoid insulting her intelligence and maturity again and to examine whether I was doing the same thing with other graduate students. That cleared the air for us to do more work. Working with clients is a two-way learning experience.

I remembered a fundamental parenting principle: age appropriateness. You don't give a bicycle to a three-year-old, and you don't provide a tricycle for a ten-year-old. You match the task to the child's developmental stage. When taking a history, ask yourself what you can reasonably expect from your client. Remember that inappropriately helping can also infantilize, just as expecting too much can overwhelm the client.

It is reasonable for clients to want effective therapy despite time constraints.

It is realistic for clients to expect a careful, competent, and caring therapist who listens. However, suppose your situation does not allow you to spend enough time with your client. You may find that your prescribed medication works no better than whatever positive relationship you can cobble together in your limited time.

When pressed for time, it is even more critical to give what my US Public Health Service boss, Dr. Cliff Culp, described as an "empathic gift." What you say reflects your understanding of what the client is expressing about their experience. It might be as simple as restating what they just told you. Saying that connects the various elements they just presented. Your comments show that their meaning has gotten through to you, and you care enough to listen closely.

Therapists' vacations are particularly challenging for dependent clients.

Vacations affect the client-therapist interaction. When you go on vacation, have a competent person on call for you and a mechanism for letting clients know how to contact them. Alert the on-call person to the clients of particular concern to you. In your original orientation with clients, tell them how to reach you. These are realistic expectations for the client to have.

That said, clients can experience your vacations as abandonment. Besides the medical-legal risks associated with perceived abandonment, your vacations may result in clients experiencing regression. That is, exhibiting behaviors they had earlier outgrown. The regression may be a warning that the client is not as close to being ready to end therapy as you'd been thinking. It is not unusual for clients to miss a session after a therapist's planned absence as a way of unconsciously saying that two can play at this game of abandonment.

Hearing so often about losses
can desensitize therapists.

A supervisor told my resident group that if they ever wondered whether they had become numb or insensitive to their clients, they should go away on vacation. He said they would notice how much more sensitive they were to what their clients said during their first couple of days back.

You will spend many hours hearing about your clients' losses and being reminded of your own. Rather than standing out, a loss can feel almost routine to you. That is not at all the case for the client. They will not be comforted by you quickly saying that you understand or reflexively voicing a platitude.

Some loss is unfathomable.

When an astronaut talks about the unique experience of feeling weightless, only other astronauts who have been weightless understand precisely what it feels like.

The same is true of losing a child. If you have not lost a child, you have no idea. Telling a grieving parent that you understand is dismissive and may make them angry.

Instead, to augment your work and acknowledge that you do not understand, you could refer the client to Compassionate Friends, a national support group for grieving, where others have lost a child. Without hugging them, you can show with the solemn softness of your speech, your reverence, and the gentleness of your manner that you know they are hurting now and may feel fragile.

The experience of loss varies with the nature of what was lost.

There are many facets to the loss of a person. A short list might include the services, income, and goods the person provided. There is also the status associated with the person. Companionship, the simple joy of being with them, and the opportunity for love and intimacy may all be lost. The futures of children and other family members are altered.

If the person left behind was the caretaker, their role and purpose are lost. If the loss was from suicide, there may be a complex mixture of feelings, depending on the nature of the lost relationship.

Sometimes, a loss is shaped by how the person who was lost made the survivor feel. For instance, imagine your client is a number. Say number 4. If a number 9 stands next to the 4, your client feels like a 94. They can feel more empowered than they did when they were standing alone. When they lose that 9, they feel like there is a gaping hole in them where the number 9 was. It's like they lost a part of themselves.

But what if a -9 stands next to them? The client feels like a -94. In that case, not having the -9 may bring relief from being free of the person who fostered the client's negative self-image. That relief could also make the client feel guilty about their happiness coming from another's misfortune.

Sometimes, when the lost person was abusive, the survivor has such intense mixed feelings that they may be at risk for regression and flashbacks. If the client has not disclosed the abuse, their intense reaction to the loss may be a clue that the person lost was an abuser.

Some losses are not straightforward. For example, a client who feels unconsciously guilty about something may feel that this guilt is partially assuaged if they have a person in their life they make sacrifices for or whose mistreatment they bear. Losing this person or situation leaves the client with what is called a "masochistic loss" because they no longer have a mechanism to help them feel that they are atoning for their mistakes.

The losses therapists hear about in therapy can come in many different forms.

As Buddhists say, life is empty of permanence but full of possibility. Death is not the only loss that is mourned. People lose jobs, partners, physical abilities, physical attractiveness, mental abilities, etc. Sometimes, getting a better job means moving and losing community. Sometimes, faith is lost. Sometimes, it is a role. I knew a former drug dealer who felt the loss of being sought and wanted by others. A person whose euphoric mania has been successfully treated may complain that they miss being euphoric.

Clients may wait their entire lives for a parent to tell them they love them. When the parent dies and never said it, there is a loss of hope that things can be different. This loss may not be as apparent, but it can have a profound effect.

As a therapist, you will not only hear about your client's losses. You will also experience the death of clients. You may sit with them through the gradual decline in their health, be with them in the hospital, or hear of their sudden death by accident, murder, or suicide.

I worked with AIDS clients when AIDS was a death sentence. As a result, I found myself wanting to live every *undeserved* minute of my life because my work reminded me how precious life is and how mortal we all are.

It can be important to understand what your client believes because having a religious faith may put loss in a different perspective for them. I write more about this and suffering in a later chapter.

At termination, therapists experience the loss of the therapeutic relationship too.

Termination of therapy accentuates the client-therapist interaction. There may be realistic reasons for therapy sessions ending, but a client's response may reflect their dynamics. They may feel like you are leaving them unfinished, with the work incomplete and them unready to handle life without you. They may experience a sense of being abandoned. If they are referred to another therapist because they're moving, they could regret having to start over again. They might wonder if the next person will be as good as or possibly better than you. They might feel grateful and proud of what they have accomplished.

Even if they knew the number of sessions they'd have with you from the beginning, they could feel rejected and wonder whether you recognized how much they needed therapy. You may see their behavior regress. If the treatment has been longer and the termination date is known, the client may recapitulate all the conflictual themes during the last few sessions. It is almost like a final reworking of the themes so they can master them.

There are many more possible responses that reflect different dynamics.

Multiple determinants go into how you feel about the termination. If things went well and the client is functioning better, you may feel like a proud parent whose efforts have resulted in your child becoming self-reliant and developing the skills that allow them to not need you. You may hope that clients will follow through with additional treatment recommendations. However, also like parents, you may worry about the skills the client still lacks and believe they are being sent out unprepared.

If the client starts the termination abruptly, you might feel misunderstood or unappreciated. You may wonder if you somehow failed the client, underestimated their resistance, or did not expect transference problems. Soul-searching, second-guessing, and "if only" thinking may follow.

Even when therapy has been effective, you can experience a kind of grief at not being able to continue with your role in the client's life. There is a bittersweet recognition that, even though you may have significantly impacted the client's life and the client recognized it, you are just a helpful bystander in the client's life. You may feel suddenly irrelevant and unneeded—like the parent with an empty nest. Hopefully, you can turn to your family or friends if you've made deposits in the support bank account to cover all those withdrawals.

A client once gave me a gift she had made herself. She told me it was so I would not forget her. I had the very same feeling about clients, wondering if I would be forgotten. I still have the gift and remember her vividly.

In private practice, I saw many clients for thirty minutes monthly, sometimes for several years. Coming from a psychoanalytical background, I always felt that the arrangement was woefully inadequate in terms of both the length and the frequency of sessions.

I felt better and less guilty when a client I had seen and terminated some years earlier saw me in the store. He told me he had gradually incorporated what we had worked on. As new life events occurred throughout the therapy, he could apply what he had been working on, knowing he would continue to be seen. He felt he could reflect on his effort in the next session. He told me he appreciated that I allowed him to be seen less frequently and for shorter sessions because he did not have to feel financial pressure to stop coming.

College students often talk about their future, just as older clients focus more on their past. When I worked with college seniors, who usually graduated in the spring, I was proud to see them complete school but sad to see them go. Imagine you had closely watched four seasons of *Friends* on TV and had to stop watching without knowing how things turned out. That approaches the nature of the loss I feel as dozens of my students graduate at the same time.

Therapists may feel defensive or tense when an event causes clients to be angry.

Perhaps treatment is not going as well as planned. Inevitably, there will be times when clients are justifiably angry with you. Again, when you are at fault, it is important to admit it. Even when you are not at fault, the situation may be a clue that you need to do more client education.

The client has also had people be mad with them. As mentioned earlier, calmly puzzling with them about the situation instead of avoiding it provides them with an example of having an open mind and curiosity. By not backing away from their criticism, you demonstrate that you, too, will examine your behaviors and the relationship. It tells them you take therapy seriously.

When a client is angry with you, it may be a splendid opportunity to comment about what is going on right then and how it relates to other patterns in their thinking and behavior.

Sometimes, clients are justifiably mad at others who may have hurt them or a loved one through mistreatment, abuse, or discrimination. If you believe this to be the case, it is helpful to validate the client. Regardless, acknowledge how they feel about it.

Sitting with your clients in their anger helps them learn to contain their affect. You aim to help them put their feelings into words instead of rage-filled acting-out behaviors. Use this opportunity to teach them techniques to calm themselves. Work to foster in them an attitude of inquisitiveness about how they came to be angry and what it means.

Even if clients are not mad at you, you may feel intensely uncomfortable in the presence of a client who is hot under the collar. If you grew up in an emotionally safe, calm environment, you may be unaccustomed to being around clients who are riled up. On the other hand, if you've been around others who were out of control, it may trigger old feelings and memories. Talking to a colleague or your own therapist may help you understand what you are experiencing.

In this chapter: I discussed how events that arise in therapy may affect the therapeutic relationship. Some events are inherent in therapy, such as ending therapy, your vacations, and length of sessions. Others, like losses and therapist mistakes, may be unexpected and evoke sadness or anger. These events are grist for the therapy mill because you may use them as teachable moments.

In the next chapter: I talk about how specific client types foster different interactions. Your particular interaction could be a clue to understanding your baffling client's type.

Chapter 19

Client Types Affect Client-Therapist Interactions

Malevolent, dependent, narcissistic, borderline, and volatile clients present unique pictures and provoke different responses from the therapist. Attractive clients, suicidal clients, and paranoid clients require the therapist to make careful decisions about how they will interact with them. The breadth of this chapter's topic is reflected in some overlaps with treatment considerations.

Malevolent clients may evoke disgust and alarm in therapists.

No one is all good or all bad. Some people, however, seem to be overcome by destructive patterns of thinking and acting that they can deny or rationalize. They so consistently behave in a destructive way that they appear evil. You may be tipped off that you are dealing with such a client when something they say revolts you or makes you feel disgusted.

You may have noticed that I have an overly optimistic view of the people I treat. And it may not fit with your experience of people in general. That is because it is rare for "evil people" to seek therapy. Sometimes, they might come as a way of showing others around them that they are good people. Their child may be referred to treatment because someone told them the child needs it, and they want to appear to be a good parent.

An evil person may come once and tell me that their partner said they would leave them if they didn't come at least once. They explain that there is nothing wrong with them. It is their partner's fault, as I should plainly see.

Instead of seeing evil people, I see their effects on others.

Scott Peck's book *People of the Lie: The Hope for Healing Human Evil* should be required reading for every therapist. There is no substitute for reading it. If you are treating a minister's wife, she may benefit from reading it as well because, in my experience, ministers' wives are often targets of evil people.

Clients' dependency needs manifest in different ways.

Clients who come across as demanding customers are more evident than clients who are more passive in their wish to be taken care of. Dependent clients are another client type that affects the therapist-client interaction because they may evoke parental feelings.

Children depend appropriately on their parents. Children have an inner drive toward autonomy, self-reliance, differentiation, and growth. In psychiatric terminology, this is called the "self-object differentiation" process. (I will never understand why the other person is called the "object.") In theory, the infant starts in "blissful symbiosis" in what is called "primary narcissism." The mother's breast is an extension of the infant. When the infant cries, they get Mom's breast, which is like the baby making their finger wiggle. The baby recognizes that they are separate from Mom only when they don't immediately get the milk. This frustration starts the process of attachment and separation.

The infant can form a secure attachment if their parents are dependable. If parenting is haphazard, the infant develops an anxious-resistant type of attachment because the infant is unsure whether the parents will understand and respond appropriately. Some infants don't seem affected by parental separation and are said to have an avoidant-attachment type of attachment.

There is an elegant description of this in John Bowlby's book *Attachment and Loss*. The current psychological literature includes further theoretical refinements.

Attachment styles carry over into later relationships, including the one with the therapist. Being taken care *of* can feel like being cared *about*. It is natural for most people to want to be taken care of. Therapists, social workers, and physicians are called "caregivers," after all.

Some clients have an anxious-resistant relationship with the therapist and feel both dependent on the therapist and yet resentful of the dependence. You may notice that they minimize their abilities and ignore their agency. They are superficially agreeable and complimentary. They discuss situations where they were passive and compliant, yet they still complain about their boss. They don't speak out because they are risk-averse and don't want to be rejected.

Clients may show considerable inertia in the process of change.

As the therapist, you may find yourself flattered and tempted to be the rescuing hero, but you may also be aware that the client is not making progress. They struggle to improve because they risk losing the secondary benefit of being sick. If they get better, they won't have a claim on your care.

Part of the difficulty with dependent clients is that they sometimes don't tell the truth, fearing you will get mad at them, not like them, or abandon them.

A client once told me I looked like George Reeves, the actor who played Superman in the original version. I asked the young woman I was going with at the time if I looked like Superman. She said, "No, you look like that nerdy Clark Kent guy who was Superman in disguise."

You might not have as obvious a sign that your client wants you to be their hero, but if you feel exceptionally skilled and unusually satisfied with yourself at the end of a session, you need to wonder if your client is dependent. You are offering the client a path to becoming self-reliant and able to leave you. The client, on the other hand, may think you don't see how genuinely needy they are. They suspect you will abandon them the first time they do something for themselves.

Remember the teenager's motto: "Never show competence." (Competence leads to more chores.) Notice that dependent clients don't disclose behaviors that reflect self-reliance or competence.

You may first notice your subtle resentment of their overdependence on you. They feel like they are ceding power to you. A somewhat analogous approach-avoidance conflict occurs when a person joins a group and wants to belong but fears being swallowed up by the group.

An even more extreme instance of this dynamic occurs when clients who idealize you want a symbiotic relationship. That wish may reflect childlike magical thinking, but it may also be a clue to psychotic, delusional thinking about you, which could lead to dangerous stalking behaviors and require intensive treatment.

There are various dynamics to explain your untrusting clients.

Untrusting client types have a pervasive negative effect on the client-therapist interaction because trust is so central to therapy. You nurture your client's trust by being reliable, doing what you say you will do, being punctual, consistently showing respect, and maintaining boundaries.

The first stage of Erik Erikson's stages of psychosocial development is trust versus mistrust. Some clients are not lucky enough to have had the kind of parents and dependable environment that creates trust. Their difficulty in trusting is a developmental difficulty that affects all their relationships to varying degrees.

Some clients developed the ability to trust and have a history of trusting people until a traumatic event occurred. They can still trust selected people, but not people who are like their abuser or in situations that are triggering. These clients are clearly victims.

Some degree of paranoid thinking is widespread, which makes the assessment even more difficult. There is a difference between paranoid clients and mistrustful clients. There are cultural influences that encourage paranoia. Politicians know people are more likely to contribute to campaigns if they are paranoid about the opposition. The media create fight-or-flight groups to promote viewership. The nightly news treats us to examples of people being victimized or overcoming victimization.

Life feels less straightforward than it was some years ago. It is more challenging to function successfully in our modern world. There is more opportunity to fail. Social media encourages us to compare our lives to the idealized lives of others. These circumstances, taken together, can make people feel like relative failures. As a result, they may want to disclaim responsibility by projecting blame onto others and seeing themselves as victims.

Paranoid clients and mistrustful clients are different. Paranoid clients' reasons for not trusting you are different from simply mistrustful clients' reasons.

The paranoid client does not trust you because they have projected their disowned motives onto you. The mistrustful client is not projecting. They don't trust you because they have not fully developed their ability to trust.

One paranoid client was happy when I shaved my beard off. He'd suspected that I had sometimes scowled at him, and he could not know for sure. He took my neutral, bearded face and projected onto me his sense of not being okay. He thought my beard was a sneaky way of hiding my opinion from him. His mistrust of me stemmed from projection. He saw himself as the victim of my devious beardedness.

Some paranoid clients will express the wish that you not let them down, like their parents and all their past therapists have. Before feeling challenged by this noble cause, ask yourself if this client may be using projection as a primary defense.

Being a righteous victim of the last therapist makes sense if the client believes they never do anything wrong. Their previous therapy was not to their liking because the previous therapist suggested they might be responsible for something the client did not like. You may need to tell them, "You are not my victim." If you are lucky enough to meet their family and they are surprisingly kinder than your client described them, that could be another sign of paranoia.

Paranoid thinking alerts you to look out for psychosis, schizophrenia, organic brain syndromes, and several other illnesses that cause paranoia. For example, demented clients often forget their keys, have their power turned off for unpaid bills, and struggle to operate the television remote. Their brain will organize their confused reality around a simple explanation: Someone else is doing all this to me.

Children whose parents are emotionally unavailable may develop pathological narcissism.

The infant starts with primary narcissism, thinking everything is part of them. When their needs are not met and they begin to experience a sense of separation, parents mitigate the situation by responding to their needs. The child becomes more self-reliant with parental support and by successfully completing incrementally more complex tasks.

At first, the child holds onto the notion of being omnipotent to avoid the terror of being helpless. As the child understands that their parents will be there for them, they can let go of some of this omnipotence. They don't need to whistle in the dark as often because they develop more confidence in themselves and their parents' support.

However, if parents are emotionally and otherwise unavailable to the child, the child will have an emptiness inside them. In reaction, they develop secondary narcissism. They can't let go of childhood omnipotence because they can count only on themselves for validation and support.

You may not get a chance to see many people with narcissistic personalities because, like the evil people I mentioned earlier, they have difficulty seeing that they need treatment. Sometimes, however, the emptiness and loneliness are so painful that they do come to treatment. In her book, *Doing Therapy: A Primer*, Dr. Gill writes:

> The therapist must become aware of the hurt child
> hiding behind the false-self and treat this hurt child

with encouragement and empathy. <u>It is this hurt child who is the real</u> patient. Treating the false-self surface is to miss the point entirely.

Underneath the grandiosity and façade of perfection, the narcissist feels like a balloon of pus. They are very vulnerable to threats to their self-esteem, which are called "narcissistic blows." You must be very gentle with narcissists and avoid popping their balloons. The work you do will take time and patience on your part. Measure your words because they are very sensitive. They expect you to soothe them the same way they soothe themselves, which is unrealistic.

They can experience anything you say as a wound because they feel it shows that you know something about them that they do not know.

When people have more than a healthy amount of narcissism, they may lack empathy, don't seem to have the same depth of emotional reaction to significant events, and may feel entitled to special treatment and attention from you and others. (Lack of empathy may also be a clue in an older client that they have frontal-temporal dementia. Look for associated signs, such as impulsivity, inappropriate social behaviors, and difficulty with language.)

You are the perfect therapist as the extension of your narcissistic client's perfect self.

The narcissistic client affects the client-therapist relationship in multiple ways. Marketing tells us we must all have the best tennis shoes, but this is particularly important to the narcissistic client because their tennis shoes are an extension of themselves. Like their therapist, their spouse and children are seen as extensions of themselves. This view fits with their need to aggrandize themselves. For example, a male narcissist may feel that dating a woman who is not beautiful reflects poorly on him. They can be a bother to attractive women.

If your client brags to others that you are the best therapist around, they are saying that, as an extension of them, you are naturally perfect too. While they may brag about you to others, they will simultaneously be very critical of you as you fail to meet their expectations of special treatment. Their children may be surprised to overhear their parents praising them to others because, at home, they are never seen as enough.

You may get a clue that you are dealing with a narcissistic client when they tell you that their illness is like no other and requires unique treatment. For example, they may have a painful condition, but it is not treatable with the usual medications because it differs from the painful conditions ordinary people have. They may claim that past therapists didn't take the extra time needed to understand how exceptionally bad the painful condition is in their unique case.

You are more likely to see the children, partners, and coworkers of narcissists.

A narcissistic parent can love and accept a child who is just like them. But the child may come to realize that their parent does not know them. If the child chooses to differentiate and become their own person, the narcissistic parent does not recognize them and devalues them. The child must choose between being idealized and unknown or being themselves and cut off. I have seen a child choose the idealized path, remain dependent on the parent, and have harmful behavior excused. The child who decides to become themselves can be successful but never do anything right in their parent's eyes. The parent may emotionally abuse or exploit their child's wish for validation.

You can find an excellent explanation of narcissism and its effect on the children of narcissists in *Children of the Self-absorbed: A Grownup's Guide to Getting Over Narcissistic Parents* by Nina Brown, EdD, LPC.

It's challenging to end a relationship with a person with pathological narcissism. Mindbodygreen has an exceptional article by Perpetua Neo, DClinPsy, on how to leave a pathological narcissist. She gives twelve tips and tells you what to expect. https://www.mindbodygreen.com/articles/breaking-up-with-a-narcissist

Clients with borderline personality disorder have fluctuating, perplexing views of the therapist. You may feel you are walking through a funhouse of mirrors that continually distorts you in different ways.

The multiple factors behind the symptoms of borderline personality disorder are beyond the scope of this book. (I will use "BPD" here to mean borderline personality disorder, not bipolar disorder.) Fortunately, these are two excellent books on the subject:

- *I Hate You Don't Leave Me: Understanding the Borderline Personality* by Jerold J. Kreisman and Hal Straus
- *Stop Walking on Eggshells: Taking Your Life Back When Someone You Care About Has Borderline Personality Disorder* by Paul T. T. Mason, MS, and Randi Kreger Mason

This article may help you understand the neuropsychiatric basis for borderline personality disorder: "The Neurobiology of Borderline Personality Disorder," by Katherine S. Pier, MD, and Lea K. Marin, MD, MPH. https://www.psychiatrictimes.com/view/neurobiology-borderline-personality-disorder

Different clients with borderline personality disorders have various degrees of difficulty with brain connections. So there are variations in the severity of symptoms.

Dialectical behavior therapy has been proven to be helpful. While there are no current specific medications available to treat BPD, I speculate that there will eventually be helpful medications that target oxytocin.

I am limiting this discussion to the reactions you might have while treating a person with BPD. The following description may resonate with your experience, even though it is both oversimplified and an overgeneralization that does not speak to the complexity of BPD.

Therapists experience compassion for the client's severe anxiety over potential abandonment and how their profound experience of loneliness and emptiness torments them.

You may feel surprised by the fluctuations in the way the client views you. These clients sometimes go quickly from idealizing and depending excessively on you to being demanding and devaluing you.

Some clients are hypersensitive and may experience interpretations as insults. They may have affective instability. They have trouble with holding a consistent mental representation of people, including a therapist, in their mind. You may feel worried about the risky, impulsive behaviors these clients show and the rage they express.

During a session, a client may express one distorted perception after another. You might feel like they are fact-checking a fast-talking political operative.

The empathy you first felt can morph into a wish to run away and a feeling of being trapped, emotionally abused, and manipulated. Sometimes, if projective identification occurs, you can inadvertently introject the client's negative projections and begin to feel their negative assessment of you is justified.

Sometimes, manipulative clients might emotionally blackmail you, threatening to hurt themselves or make rash decisions.

In this chapter: I discussed how clingy, mistrusting, malevolent, volatile, or potentially suicidal clients shape client-therapist interactions.

In the next chapter: I deal with a variety of situations that play a role in client-therapist interactions.

Chapter 20

Client Situations That Influence Client-Therapist Interactions

It is helpful to anticipate common situations in therapy. Sometimes, your client is slow to improve or is suicidal. Your client may have cancer or be volatile. Each situation affects the client-therapist relationship.

Everything that happens in therapy, including sexual attraction, is potentially relevant to the treatment.

YAVIS are **y**oung, **a**ttractive, **v**erbal, **i**ntelligent, and **s**uccessful clients. William Schofield coined the term in his book *Psychotherapy: The Purchase of Friendship*. According to Wikipedia, Schofield felt mental health professionals are biased toward these clients because they form positive relationships more easily and may be more likely to be responsive in therapy. Though a source is not apparent, there is a popular acronym for people who are the opposite of YAVIS: HOUND (**h**omely, **o**ld, **u**nsuccessful, **n**onverbal, and **d**umb).

Your treatment setting may determine which group you see more of. The YAVIS present the risk of you overlooking their weaknesses. And you might overlook the strengths of the HOUNDs.

YAVIS are more likely to respond to your treatment and give you a feeling of satisfaction. Add to this that they are also physically appealing, and you may find them sexually attractive. If you find yourself treating an attractive client, know that it is normal to be attracted to attractive people. But it can be distracting from therapy. If you find yourself having a sexual thought about a client, you might try the "monkey thoughts" approach used in meditation.

When meditating, the goal is focus on breath. But random thoughts can be distracting. The experts' advice: Think of the thoughts as clouds passing across the sky. You're not to scold yourself for thinking the thoughts. Instead, don't invest too much energy in trying not to think about them. That just gives the thoughts more energy. So, the trick is not to resist thinking the thoughts. Just let them go by and don't dwell on them.

My late first wife's mother offered wise advice before our marriage. She said there would be times when my wife would be attracted to someone, like a little bird flying through her mind. She said to let the little bird fly through, but don't build a nest.

Everything that happens in therapy is grist for the therapy mill. Having a sexual thought about a client is no different. But a recurrent sexual thought may be more than just a random thought. To determine if there's an issue, answer the following questions:

- Are you bored with what the client is talking about?
- Is the topic challenging to digest?
- Are you tired of listening to clients today?
- Is there something about this client's appearance that is like others who have been important to you?
- Are you having difficulties in your own personal relationships?

Don't assume that the client is being seductive. There are cultural pressures to dress well, and people with social skills tend to be friendly. However, if you feel you are getting multiple nonverbal cues, you must ask yourself whether the client is acting out an oedipal issue. They may be attracted to you because you are forbidden. Does the client have a history of being sexually abused or made to feel their only power or worth is in their sexuality? Does your client have a history of testing limits?

You already know you should not act on your sexual thoughts. Your knee-jerk reaction to having a sexual thought might be to become distant and formal with the client. They may see this in your nonverbal behavior and experience it as a rejection of them as a person.

A research project asked shoppers to respond to ethical situations. Then the shoppers went into the store and made multiple decisions about buying grocery items. They had to resist their buying impulses. The researchers then asked them to respond to similar ethical situations. The finding: Shoppers were not as ethical after having shopped. In the course of your day, you will have to make multiple clinical judgments. Like the shoppers, your judgment may be affected by fatigue from having to make so many.

If you recognize that your life circumstances make you vulnerable to your sexual attraction to a client, consider seeing that client in the morning when you are ethically fresh. Talk to your supervisor, colleague, or therapist. Add structure. Remember that you could consider referring the client to another therapist. Don't underestimate the power of countertransference feelings.

I did not realize how often therapy has some low-grade, never-discussed sexual tension in the background until I began working with lesbians. They found it easier to be forthright and open with me because they did not care how I saw them sexually. I also felt more relaxed because I did not feel my appearance was being assessed.

When I saw students remotely due to COVID, I noticed that young women who had been sexually abused talked about it with me more easily because we were never in the same room.

A client may dress better when they are getting over their depression. You may unnecessarily worry that it is a sign of sexual attraction.

Your clients could be the object of emotional blackmail.

A client might insist that their child get a job or leave. The child may then try to make their parent feel guilty about having a homeless child who has no means of support.

You will hear that a client's partner threatened to kill themselves if your client leaves them.

Your middle-aged clients will relate that their widowed parents constantly make them feel guilty about not being present to help them.

College graduates will complain they are being shamed for accepting a job far from their parents' home.

Susan Forward and Donna Frazier discuss emotional blackmail and how to deal with it in their book *Emotional Blackmail: When the People in Your Life Use Fear, Obligation, and Guilt to Manipulate You*.

Clients who appear volatile in the session require special considerations.

Another situation that affects the client-therapist interaction is the client who might need involuntary treatment. Clients worry you will commit them involuntarily, refer them to a doctor who will poison their brain and body, reveal their secrets, exert devious power over them, waste their money, or subject them to stigma just because they're seen in your office.

Clients who are paranoid due to their psychotic process are terrified and may strike out in defense. They likely are not inherently violent.

Sometimes, clients fear themselves. They fear their violent impulses. You may sense that they don't want to awaken the sleeping lion and tiptoe through the interview when they speak unusually softly and carefully.

Try to not behave in any way that might seem intimidating. Here are some useful tips:

- Do not stand over your client.
- Make yourself seem smaller. Slouch! Remove an oversized coat.
- Offer them something to drink, but make sure they see you open it so they know you have not drugged it.
- Offer them something to eat that comes in a package.
- Keep out of arm's reach and don't invade their body space.
- Don't raise your voice.
- Make friends first with nonthreatening, superficial conversation.
- If possible, arrange the furniture in advance so they don't feel cornered but you can get out without getting past them.
- Explain what you are going to do before you do it.
- Don't turn your back on them.
- Make sure others are in the vicinity.

Sometimes, you will be the one who is fearful of violence. Seeing a client in a jail or prison setting requires planning. While all prisoners may have broken the law, not everyone is a sociopath. Some are there for nonviolent crimes. Some violated the law because of their mental illness, addiction, or both. You are unlikely to know that during a first encounter.

It is safer not to trust that they are being honest with you or can control their impulses. Avoid wearing anything a client could use to choke you. Wear drab clothing that covers your body and does not reveal your shape. Your shoes should not slow your movement. Give anything sharp to someone to hold for you.

While having a guard with you might restrict conversation, you should weigh the risks and ask the guard what they think. If the client is in shackles, the shackles are there for a reason. Find out as much as possible about the client before seeing them. Guards can be valuable sources of corroborating information.

Clients voicing suicidal thoughts during sessions trigger the helicopter therapist in me.

When a client is potentially suicidal, the intensity of the client-therapist relationship can rise.

You have heard of helicopter parents who hover over their kids and overprotect them. When I have a client who may be at risk for suicidal behavior, I find myself having to resist the impulse to become a hypervigilant, helicopter psychiatrist.

With every client, I try to make a point of thinking about the acronym PODS: **p**sychotic, **o**rganic, **d**rug-affected/**d**epressed, and **s**uicidal. I look for clues that the client might have a latent psychosis, a drug-induced psychosis, or a chronic psychotic illness. I search for signs of a physical disease that could be behind their presentation or may be contributing to it. I watch for signs of depression and illicit drug/medication problems. Most importantly, I ask myself about the risk of suicide and/or violence. If I don't expect the unexpected, I may not see it until it's too late.

It would not be unusual to feel threatened when there is a chance that your client may kill themselves. Assessing suicidal risk is complicated and problematic. While demographics can somewhat predict the long-term risk factors for suicide, many people believe it is impossible to say with certainty whether someone will kill themselves in the short run.

Most people would agree that the best predictor of future suicidal attempts is the history of a past one. Look for risk factors like age, being unemployed, being a Caucasian male, recent loss, history of bipolar disorder, history of autism, history of borderline personality, and history of impulsivity. I suspect that some risk factors incorporated in age-related risk have to do with chronic pain, multiple chronic illnesses, loss of function, loss of purpose/status associated with work, and loss of family members.

I have found that, for young people in particular, a sense of rejection and alienation from family is a powerful push toward suicidal behavior. That alienation contrasts with the acceptance and love the client may feel awaits them in the idyllic afterlife, which others have unknowingly made dangerously attractive.

When you see a distraught client suddenly be at peace, that is the time to worry and inquire. When people have made up their minds to kill themselves, they don't worry about their dire situation. You may discover that they are giving away their possessions.

Confidentiality and the Health Insurance Portability and Accountability Act (HIPAA) restrictions sometimes make getting information and communications tricky, if not almost impossible. Still, it would be best to have a team of people to treat and monitor the suicidal client effectively. Getting information from the family and the client is vital since the client may be reluctant to discuss past attempts. Clients who do not speak about their suicidal thoughts are said to have high lethality. Enlist roommates, family members, trusted religious leaders, etc.

Please don't assume that the family grasps how bad it is. Also, don't let the client's protest that the family does not care about them stop you from convincing the client to let you talk to them in front of the client. I have often been surprised at how distorted the client's view of family was.

Depressed clients tend to feel like the family is unchangeable, just like everything else they are struggling with. Don't let their sense of helplessness become your sense of helplessness. Remember that you have the option of committing them if they can be found to be a danger to themselves or others.

Earlier, I mentioned frantic hopelessness as a significant risk factor and talked about the need to reduce anxiety and agitation quickly.

Addressing sleep problems is also vital. As mentioned earlier, time passes slowly when a client lies alone in bed without diversion. And that gives them time to ruminate. Some research suggests people are more likely to have suicidal thoughts at night. You can reduce suicidal risk if you can get the client calm and asleep.

Addressing the sleep problem may require you to push others to get the client in with a prescriber if you don't prescribe. Under-medicating in this situation can be risky.

Clients have told me that they tried to kill themselves only five minutes after having the first suicidal thought. That makes it vital for you to reduce opportunities. Have family members remove and lock weapons. Get them to remove knives, rope, or car keys that can be used in a suicide attempt.

Know how many days of your prescribed medication are lethal, and don't prescribe more than that at a time. Ask family or friends to hold and dispense the medicines. Remind clients that if they stop medications prematurely, their symptoms of depression will likely come back.

Make sure they and their family know how to reach you. Have good call coverage. Don't neglect client and family education. Let them know about the resources and support groups available. Get it across to them that it takes time for medication to work and that there will be ups and downs.

Infrequently, you will find a client who has inherited a problem with the serotonin transporter (SERT). That client is likely to become extremely suicidal if placed on selective serotonin reuptake inhibitors (SSRIs) or other medications that raise serotonin. If you suspect this is the case, you must stop the medication quickly, protect the client, and do genetic testing before proceeding. GeneSight tests for serotonin transporter gene problems.

The complex role of the multiple types of serotonin receptors in brain and body function is beyond the scope of this book. But I have found three technical articles that may be helpful:

- An article in *Neurochemistry International* by V. Sreeja and others: "Pharmacogenetics of selective serotonin reuptake inhibitors (SSRI): A serotonin reuptake transporter (SERT) based approach." https://www.sciencedirect.com/science/article/abs/pii/S0197018623002000
- "The Expanded Biology of Serotonin," an article by M. Berger and others in the *Annual Review of Medicine*: https://pmc.ncbi.nlm.nih.gov/articles/PMC5864293/
- "Serotonin Transporter Gene Polymorphisms and Selective Serotonin Reuptake Inhibitor Tolerability: Review of Pharmacogenetic Evidence," an article in *Pharmacotherapy* by Zhu and others: https://pubmed.ncbi.nlm.nih.gov/28654193/

Some clients have good ego strength and have functioned despite the growing physical and mental changes associated with depression. When these people come to treatment, the depressive process is advanced, and they are considerably more miserable than their functioning would suggest. It may look like time is not running out, but it is.

The public thinks of depression as severe sadness and difficulty enjoying things. But as it progresses, there are more changes in the way the depressed person thinks. I would say there is a narrowing of thought. It becomes more challenging for the client to consider alternatives to suicide. It becomes increasingly difficult to see the positive in things or believe that anything can change for the better. If the client develops psychotic depression, don't forget that electroconvulsive therapy (ECT) was at one time the treatment of first choice and is still done.

The quality of depression in bipolar illness feels different to me. It is darker, more malignant, gripping, and disabling. It is the monster under the bed. Treating it may require multiple medications, some of which have significant side effects. Bipolar depression feels like the stage IV cancer of depression, and the drugs that treat it feel like chemotherapy. You wouldn't tell the client not to have chemotherapy if it is going to save their life. Neither should you neglect to use lifesaving medications that are designed to treat bipolar disorder and may risk significant side effects.

Consider lithium, which has been shown to reduce suicidal ideas even at low doses. It is not advertised because it is so inexpensive. Learn more in SK Sarai, HM Mekala, and S Lippmann's article titled "Lithium Suicide Prevention: A Brief Review and Reminder" in *Innovations in Clinical Neuroscience*: https://pmc.ncbi.nlm.nih.gov/articles/PMC6380616/

I don't worry about being manipulated by a client threatening suicide. I worry about not taking them seriously enough. But there is a catch-22 when you have a client at risk for suicide. You need to believe in yourself and that you can do the right thing, but that sense of being empowered also makes you feel responsible for the outcome. Share your concerns and decision-making with your colleagues.

Even with all the support systems in place and the client adequately treated with a medication that has helped others, I sometimes find myself holding my breath until the client shows signs of getting significantly better or is hospitalized. At times like these, I count on my family to understand that I am preoccupied with something I can't discuss. As they give me nonspecific support and understanding, I am making withdrawals from the family emotional support bank account. Then I will make a deposit in the family bank account as soon as possible.

> **When I commit a client to involuntary inpatient treatment, I feel an intense need to control what I can because I have started a process that may fail.**

You may need to take a medical/legal risk and commit a client involuntarily because you fear they may harm themselves or others. This situation may test the collaborative nature of the client-therapist interaction. You want to document your reasoning, all the options you considered, how you conferred with others, and the information you based your decision on. Getting the client's permission to include their family in the decision process is good.

Avoid letting the family transport the client to the hospital. Clients may convince the family that they don't need to go. They may jump out of the car. The client's transport and waiting time before being admitted to the hospital may take many hours, even a day, and clients will benefit from any packaged snacks you can give them to eat during their wait.

Follow up to ensure that the information reaches the staff treating your client. Somebody may not forward your information from the emergency department to the receiving hospital. A client could change their story. They could be prematurely released because there is no document to tell the new assessor what you knew when you originally determined the danger.

The ultimate decision about involuntary commitment rests with the doctor at the emergency receiving facility. You may feel a small measure of comfort that there is a fail-safe in case you overestimated the danger. When you fill out an involuntary commitment form, you are merely asking law enforcement to take your client to be evaluated, and you are stating that you have found evidence to suggest that the client has said or done things in the last thirty days (the number of days may vary from state to state) that have led you to believe they are a danger to themselves or others.

In most states, a hospitalized client will be released within seventy-two hours if the hospital cannot prove to a hearing officer that they should stay longer.

Before informing your client of your decision, make sure you have adequate staff to prevent the client from suddenly running out of your office. The client should remain in your sight until law enforcement arrives. Waiting with the client for law enforcement to come can feel painfully long.

I am sometimes surprised that once I've made the decision, the client relaxes. Deep down, they realize they need more intensive help. Depending on the client's state of mind, I may offer some positives about inpatient treatment and assure them that I will be available for follow-up treatment after their discharge. I may try to address some of the common misconceptions about psychiatric hospitals.

Know what HIPAA conditions will allow you to communicate with future providers. You will also need to understand the Tarasoff laws concerning your obligation to notify intended victims of violence.

The following are some useful resources:

- Colorado State University has a website with warning signs, links to other resources, and assessment tools: https://health.colostate.edu/suicide-prevention/
- *Clinical Manual for the Assessment and Treatment of Suicidal Patients* by Dr. John Chiles et al. https://psychiatryonline.org/doi/book/10.1176/appi.books.9781615378982
- *Stronger than Death* by Sue Chance
- *Choosing to Live: How to Defeat Suicide Through Cognitive Therapy* by Thomas E. Ellis
- The National Suicide Hotline: 1-800-273-8255
- The Transgender Suicide Prevention Hotline: 1-877-565-8860
- The American Association of Suicidology: https://suicidology.org/
- The American Foundation for Suicide Prevention: https://afsp.org/about-afsp/
- Suicide Prevention Resource Center: https://sprc.org/
- The Virtual Helpbox App: https://www.research.va.gov/research_in_action/Virtual-Hope-Box-smartphone-app-to-prevent-suicide.cfm

Initially, when therapy is going nowhere, it can be both frustrating and motivating.

In *The Little Prince*, the little prince tries unsuccessfully to tame the fox. In frustration, he finally asks the fox what he can do to tame him. The fox says the little prince must waste time with him, and then the fox will allow himself to be tamed.

I have been reminded of this so many times when working with clients. Wasted time is not wasted. For example, you may spend time getting nowhere, such as trying one medication after another. By persisting, you show your belief that something will eventually work out. It shows the client that you care enough to take on a frustrating task and that you believe in their future.

Seeing you persist despite the apparent lack of progress may inspire clients to keep trying as well. Ruby K. Payne tells the story of a child who comes home with one A and the rest F's on their report card. When asked why they worked hard to get an A in one class, the child explained that they liked the teacher. Sometimes, clients will work hard to improve, even when nothing has worked out for them, because they like you (Payne 2018).

Frustrated therapists recognize that an unsatisfying situation is just the beginning.

To digress for a moment, I would like to elaborate on how dissatisfaction is a necessary but insufficient cause of therapeutic progress. Here is a quote from the book my wife and I wrote, *Search: A Guide for College Life*:

Mike Rutherford–Rutherford Learning Group https://www.rutherfordlg.com/—has said that dissatisfaction alone is not enough for someone, or some group, to make changes and overcome their natural resistance to making changes. A person needs to feel a heightened sense of dissatisfaction and then be introduced to an interesting vision of what things would be like if they made changes. That is not enough. He feels that helping them make the first successful small steps towards change is a crucial part of the equation. From a talk we could hear, here is his equation:

Dissatisfaction+ interesting Vision+ Successful first small steps> Resistance= Change Roquemore (2020)

When a client presents to you, they already have some dissatisfaction. Working with them to develop their interesting vision is part of Mike Rutherford's equation for change, which involves hope. I have found that working with the client to imagine the first small steps and the concrete details of those steps increases their chance of having hope. It shows them how to turn their hope into action (Rutherford 2014).

I want to use Alcoholics Anonymous (AA) to illustrate these concepts further because AA has all the ingredients of Mike Rutherford's equation for change. In AA, the alcoholic's sponsor spends untold, often frustrating, time with the alcoholic as they go through the difficulties of their daily struggle to sustain sobriety. The sponsor demonstrates their belief in their sponsee and uses AA's recovery program to provide concrete steps.

Hearing other members discussing their recovery paints a vivid picture of recovery that helps the alcoholic come to see how remarkable recovery is. It becomes something the alcoholic wants more than alcohol. In the open meetings I have been able to attend, I have found something sacred in the atmosphere of acceptance, forgiveness, and redemption there. AA believes, as do I, that "dis-ease," or "un-ease," has physical, mental, and spiritual components. AA welcomes the prodigal son home.

Don't underestimate your contribution when clients are making progress.

Mother Teresa was quoted as saying, "Not all of us can do great things. But we can do small things with great love."

Sometimes, doing a small thing can make a difference in someone's life. At times, you may feel your light may be small. But even a little light may shine brightly in someone's great darkness. In your client's great darkness, you could be the first person to take the time to listen, show compassion, or believe in them.

Think about how many times you have heard a prominent person who grew up in adversity talk about how much it meant to see their grandmother's face light up when they came into the room and how much their grandmother believed in them when no one else did. Maybe a teacher saw something in them for the first time. Children can be like weeds that shoot roots out to find water from other sources when their soil is dry, or like trees whose branches reach toward the sun. Your profession gives you an opportunity to offer that water and light.

When your client is at risk of dying from cancer or by suicide, you may feel unusual pressure to provide hope.

When the client has cancer, this is another situation that has a bearing on therapist-client interactions. Therapists know that hopeful cancer patients are more likely to conscientiously follow treatment recommendations. Cancer clients at first may hope to be cured. If that seems less likely, they hope for a shorter-term goal, like having less pain or living long enough to celebrate a particular event. You may feel it is not so much the thing hoped for as the act of hoping itself that is necessary.

Despite knowing how central hope is to their client's well-being, it can be hard to foster hope when you feel realistically discouraged about your client's future.

Having limited time with the client can feel analogous to eating an ice cream cone. The ice cream tastes even better because there is only so much of it. Yet that knowledge sometimes interferes with our ability to savor it.

Focusing the client on the small victories and milestones can contribute to a more positive atmosphere. Lori Hope wrote a book that helps family and friends understand how to support a cancer patient. It is titled *Help Me Live: 20 Things People with Cancer Want You to Know.*

Helping suicidal clients get past their narrow thinking about future possibilities can be life-saving. Changing their thinking begins the process of them discovering a persuasively positive vision of the future, along with the concrete, small steps to achieve it.

Enlisting the client's family may help you feel less alone in your task of providing hope. Sometimes, when you've enlisted them in the effort, the family emerges as the source of acceptance, forgiveness, and redemption the client needs.

In this chapter: I discussed situations that play a role in client-therapist interactions, such as having an attractive client, a suicidal client, a volatile client, a client who is making slow progress, or a client with cancer.

In the next series of chapters: My primary focus is on dynamics and how they affect the way the client sees themselves and relates to others. The trap of self-development is also mentioned. The next chapter will also discuss the role hormones and joint hypermobility may play in dynamics.

Part 3

UNDERSTANDING CLIENT DYNAMICS

The motivation for clients' behavior is multi-determined. Family, culture, abuse, sex, addiction, parenting, work, and physical illness all shape client behaviors.

This section examines how your client's dynamics play out in affairs, family relationships, and work. It mentions some unusual abuse dynamics and sexual behaviors that are not about sex. Understanding your baffling client's dynamics could be the key to understanding what makes them tick.

Chapter 21

Dynamics That Involve Just the Client

This chapter mentions clients who present as self-satisfied. It discusses clients whose dynamics are affected by hormonal or connective tissue problems.

There are clients whose personal dynamics illustrate Freud's well-known psychodynamic formulations that correspond to the way the nervous system develops: the oral, anal, phallic, and oedipal stages. Rather than elaborate on those dynamics, I want to address a dilemma associated with self-development.

Your task is to focus on the client's self, helping them grow less self-centered. You aim to help them develop their self-knowledge and self-acceptance so they are freed up to invest in others and a purpose outside themselves.

Sometimes, clients mistakenly believe the purpose of therapy is to make them more self-satisfied.

Clients may believe your job is to make them satisfied with who they currently are and make them more successful at doing the same maladaptive things they are doing now. They want to be a less depressed, less anxious version of themselves. Having loving kindness for oneself is essential, but they want to be absolved of any responsibility in their current situation.

In Oscar Wilde's play *Lady Windermere's Fan: A Play About a Good Woman*, Wilde has the character Dumby say, "There are only two tragedies. One is not getting what one wants, and the other is getting it."

When the self-centered man attains his heart's desire, he is like a greyhound on the racetrack that catches the mechanical rabbit. The satisfaction can feel brief, and the purpose can feel illusory.

The other problem with succeeding is that reality is characterized by impermanence. Personal success is fleeting. Beauty ages. Fortunes are lost. Achievements seem less relevant over time.

As mentioned earlier, because things are empty of constancy, they are full of possibility. However, that leads to insecurity and frustration for the part of us that wants ground under our feet.

(Pema Chodron addresses this eloquently in her discussion of the concept of *shenpa* in her book *Don't Bite the Hook:*

Finding Freedom from Anger, Resentment and Other Destructive Emotions.)

Clients may not get the dead-end quality of self-pursuit. They think your job is to make them better, not different.

Part of the paradox of self-development is that both you and the client must focus on the client's self to understand it as part of their moving on to become less self-conscious and start connecting more with others.

Over time, a parallel process is happening to you as a therapist. As you understand yourself better and feel more confident, you can be less self-conscious. And that frees you up to see more clearly what is happening in the therapy right before you.

A family therapist trainer once said it is easy to work with someone off the street, throw them in with a family therapy situation, and have them pick up the family dynamics and interact therapeutically with the family. He said it was harder to work with someone who already had a professional identity and was too self-conscious to see what was happening in the session. Whether or not we have an established professional identity, we all must start from where we are now.

Altered hormones may be behind the dynamics.

When examining dynamic theories, it is easy to overlook the fact that the client has a physical body. Sometimes, that body is a driving force in behavior.

I remember two adult brothers who had frustrated the clinic staff. Each was found to have extreme passivity. And each of their therapists felt they could not get them to do anything. The brothers seemed content to play video games, and they were not interested in losing weight, dating, or working. When they were tested for hypogonadism and found to have deficient testosterone, their problems with drive activity made more sense.

Changes in female hormones can affect the brain as well.

I once looked at the age all my female patients were when they first came into treatment. I found the median age was thirty-seven. That is when women may be coping with children, partners, aging parents, jobs, money, and responsibilities. The cumulative effect of those stressors could easily explain why thirty-seven is the median age. But it is also an age associated with perimenopause. Variations in estrogen metabolism affect the brain. Just scanning this complex article may give you an idea of the importance of estrogen in brain function: "Estrogen effects on the brain: actions beyond the hypothalamus via novel mechanisms" by Bruce S. McEwen et al. https://www.ncbi.nlm.nih.gov/pmc/articles/PMC3480182/

Connective tissue disorders can play a surprising role in dynamics.

If a client has problems with the integrity of their connective tissue, they may be unstable when standing and feel wobbly. This sensation can be subtle. They may become anxious without connecting physical unsteadiness with the anxiety. I have had several clients whose first presentation was a kind of generalized anxiety. Further workup revealed postural orthostatic tachycardia syndrome (POTS), Ehlers-Danlos syndrome, joint hypermobility syndrome (JHS), or some combination of these. When you see a person who is anxious and does not have the usual anxiety disorder dynamics, think about these illnesses.

Sometimes, the client finds an unexpected solution to their problem.

One client, who was a husband and father, had used his back pain as a way to avoid various responsibilities. This secondary gain was okay with him until his wife told him he shouldn't stress his back by having intercourse. He had painted himself into a corner. Two sessions later, he announced that his back was healed. He had heard about a tent meeting in town featuring a faith healer. So he'd gone down and been healed.

When I was a psychiatric resident on call, I admitted a woman who was assisted into the admissions office by family members holding her on both sides. They explained that she had lost her vision, and her family doctor thought it was all in her head. I was already tired and had a lot more work ahead of me. I took down some basics and did the physical without thinking much about it.

When I got to the eye exam, I pulled up her eyelids to look at the blood vessels in the back of her eyes. She proclaimed, "I can see!" I said it was great and finished the physical. I did not check the next day to see if the cure had stuck, but conversion symptoms are seldom straightforward.

In this chapter: I talked about physical issues that may be impacting your client.

In the next chapter: I will cover sexual dynamics.

Chapter 22

Uncovering Baffling Sexual Dynamics

Multiple determinants go into sexual behaviors, and it is important to avoid drawing premature conclusions about them.

Sexual behaviors may not be primarily about sexual drive.

My experience working with teenagers and college students has taught me how vulnerable young women can be.

One of the most poignant examples of vulnerability was Sandra, a sixteen-year-old girl who had recently transferred to another high school because of her reputation for promiscuity. Her modest dress and pleasant appearance made her look wholesome rather than sexual. But Sandra didn't know much about sex, didn't have much sexual drive, and didn't find the sex act enjoyable.

She did eventually identify a vicious cycle. She would feel worthless and unlovable. A boy would flirt with her. Then she'd begin to believe she could be cared for. Sandra would do anything the boy wanted her to do sexually. For a brief moment, she'd feel wanted, desirable, and loved. She'd so rarely felt that and would have so much hope associated with it that when she realized she had been complicit in being used, it was all the more devastating. She felt betrayed and degraded. She had been fooled and abandoned once more. Her self-loathing was intense. She resolved not to be fooled again.

The boy would talk to his peers, who would speak to their girlfriends. The girls at the school were fearful of her taking away their boyfriends, so they ostracized her. It felt like everyone knew, and people at school would shy away from her. This situation made Sandra feel even more needy for validation. And this set her up to give in to the next boy. When a person is emotionally starving for love, validation, and acceptance, they are at risk of being exploited.

In my work with children and teens in a residential treatment center, I worked with children who were perpetrators of sexual abuse. I found it hard to believe that, at eleven years old, a child could be a sexual predator. One child was very skilled at spotting other children who had been abused and who could become their victims. They could identify the one abused child in a room of sixty potential victims.

Sometimes, revenge, the excitement of the forbidden, or competitive strivings are the motives behind what appear on the surface to be simply sexually motivated behaviors.

For example, some men have mothers who were cold and unsatisfied with anything their children did when growing up. These men find themselves seducing women and leading them on, unaware that their motive is to let them down. It is not the sex they seek but the opportunity to turn the tables on the women and make them feel they are not enough, just like their mother made them feel when they were children.

Clients' interpersonal dynamics may manifest in their sexual behaviors.

Nowhere are dynamics more reductionist than when we try to understand the motives behind some sexual behaviors. Nonetheless, I will describe some of the dynamics that I believe were behind affairs.

Different sexual needs may be the dynamic behind some affairs. For example, clients have explained that sometimes, they want their partner to be tender and loving, and other times, they want passionate, lusty sex that does not make time for tenderness. One may have an affair when the other is consistently absent from their sexual relationship.

Ernesto's difficulty with being able to love resulted in an affair.

Having never experienced love or seen examples of it, Ernesto did not know how to love or form an intimate attachment. He equated the initial, perhaps pheromone-driven, infatuation with mature love. Ernesto fell in love with the idea of love. When infatuation stopped, the need for joint everyday problem-solving began. He could not build the give-and-take, interdependent caring about each other that loses "me "and "you" in favor of "us." Having sex did not grow into making love. Emotional intimacy eluded Ernesto, and he was stuck with sex without love.

Habituation became a problem for Ernesto. Habituation is seen in different situations. For example, when a person repeatedly views pornography, the stimulus that is initially exciting grows less exciting over time. The viewer needs to seek something novel to achieve the same level of excitement. Then they become habituated to the new stimulus, and so on.

Ernesto had an affair and explained to himself that it was because his sex life had become routine. Because he was just having sex, he had become habituated. The enduring emotional intimacy that would have sustained him and given him relationship depth was missing. He and his partner lacked the contentment that can serve as a buffer against the difficulties associated with the ups and downs of sexual performance and life.

There are other people who don't become unfaithful; they never were faithful to begin with. They are not capable of fidelity. The cause may be a lack of impulse control. Other people may be unable to form attachments. Perhaps they are sociopaths who marry for money or political advancement.

Some people marry to convince themselves that they are not gay or lesbian, but it does not work. They have difficulty ignoring their sexuality and may have an affair. Their partners may feel unattractive and seek reassurance outside the relationship as well. Often, there is more love between the couple than there is in the average marriage, along with a basis for a friendship that lasts beyond the divorce. Both parties may have a long history of kindness toward each other and want the best for each other, but the process is still painful and confusing to the kids.

The dynamics of naivete and overconfidence may lead to an affair.

I once heard a minister deliver a sermon on adultery. He said that an affair dilutes or adulterates the energy necessary for a relationship. He spoke about how naive people overestimate their impulse control and put themselves in situations that set them up to give in.

I have taken advantage of his concept of stages to talk to people dealing with impulse control. The minister said it starts with a look at an attractive person. At that point, if the person looking is aware of the process, this is when it's easiest to change the behavior—to look away and try to think about something else.

Next comes the lust stage, in which the person allows themselves to develop fantasies about the object of their attention.

In the lingering stage, the person will create a way to be around the attractive person. In the lingering stage, they trust their impulse control and tell themselves it is just an innocent interaction.

In the lure stage, the two people find themselves in a more seductive situation, alone and lacking deterrents to acting on their impulses. Then, the impulse is acted on. It seems the act happened suddenly, but both parties ignored the warning signs that would have made it easier to prevent it.

I've had several clients who could relate to this situation. They told me that work compounded the temptations by throwing them and the other party together on work projects, where they worked long hours. That tired them out, lowered their impulse control, and isolated them. At other times, work resulted in employees being assigned away from home for extended periods.

Dahlia's husband's affair extricated her from a loveless marriage.

Dahlia had come to understand that leaving her dysfunctional husband would make her life much easier, but it would take time, energy, and money. She had just enough to hold things together and take care of her kids. She lacked the added energy needed for transformation. Even if her religious beliefs had allowed her, she was too tired to have an affair.

When Dahlia met her husband, she'd felt needed. She mistakenly equated that with being loved. But over time, she felt used. She was ambivalent about the idea of leaving her husband, but she convinced herself that there were some things she could do to improve her life without committing herself to making that decision. Having a plan made her more optimistic, even though there was no immediate relief in sight.

She set about getting more education, finding a better job, saving money, and getting her kids through school. Dahlia was not a manipulative person. I doubt it occurred to her that her diminished sexual interest would lead her husband to have an affair. But, over time, it did. Then Dahlia could justify a divorce. And by that time, she was prepared. She felt his affair just happened, but it was actually the culmination of an unconscious war of attrition.

Some affair dynamics revolve around affirmation. Men have told me that their wives belittled them in public and demeaned them sexually in private. These men found a "testimonial woman" to have an affair with until they could feel good enough about themselves to leave their abusive wives.

I have treated testimonial women who rehabilitated men, only to be left for less nurturing but more physically attractive women. I suspect that the nurturing and mothering these women provided turned these men off because men want a partner, not a mother.

There are also baffling sexual dynamics related to actual inadequacy. Women have often complained of having to over-function and mother their inadequate, dependent husbands who refused to grow up. Their sex life suffered in part because these women did not want to sleep with a "son," and the men did not want to sleep with a "mother." When I hear this part of the story, I am listening for any clue that the inadequate husband slept with a victim in the vicinity, like a child or the wife's best friend. Some men are too lazy or inadequate to pick up someone at a bar or seek someone online.

Some affair dynamics involve a client's unwillingness to lose marital advantages. Clients may have convinced themselves that they loved a partner who offered them and their kids security and kindness, only to realize later that it was need and not love. They find the partner does not excite them sexually or romantically. Rather than end the marriage and lose their security, they have an affair.

Men have told me they stopped caring about their relationship with their wives years before the divorce. It did not matter if a wife learned how to communicate better, was more appreciative, offered sex more, or understood the husband better.

It took me a while to realize that when I was treating the wives of these men, I was wasting the wives' money trying to help them communicate better. But sometimes, a wife needed to make that effort before she could believe she had tried everything. Then she could drop her denial, grieve, and regain agency over her future. Some baffling sexual dynamics involve affair dynamics in which an unconscious contract is broken. I have not seen many trophy wife couples, but I believe these marriages are in trouble if the wife gains weight or the husband loses money. If the relationship develops into a meaningful, loving one over time, the trophy wife must adapt to becoming a nurse to her much older mate.

I treated an older man who had dominated and mistreated his younger wife over the years. The wife's life and family situation prevented her from leaving. She was unusually fit, and it seemed she had decided that staying healthy and outliving him would ultimately give her a life of her own. Eventually, the older man needed his wife to care for him, but she used the opportunity to withhold care as a kind of torture. When you see contempt in the eyes of your elderly male client's wife, ask yourself if he is getting his medication and the treatment he needs.

Being loved nurtures the remarkable person a partner has stunted.

Rose's partner was well known for his compassion and selfless behavior. Her partner was a genuinely good person and parent. On the other hand, Rose, who was a teacher, was seen as somewhat distant in her relationships with her colleagues. I wondered whether they felt subtly intimidated by Rose's trim figure, the understated elegance of her clothes, and her fine facial features.

Sometimes, her students' parents would ask the principal to move their children to a different class. Most students and their parents would begrudgingly acknowledge that Rose was an excellent teacher who took a special interest in needy students. But her aloofness made her seem cold.

It was a puzzle to me that Rose's partner would be so dismissive and undermine her when he was so lovely to everyone else. Eventually, I learned that his mother gave him up as a small child. And he took out his anger on Rose. She tried many things but found her character being subtly attacked daily. She described it as soul-destroying.

Rose described her affair as lifesaving. What baffled me the most was how she almost became another person. Others noticed a warmth and openness they had not seen before in Rose. She was not just in love; she had discovered that she could be loved and valued for herself.

I felt sad that two good people couldn't get along, but I was blown away by how much a person can blossom when they're loved and how that person had been there all along, pushed down inside. It was like love had melted the iciness.

Eventually, Rose left her partner, and it felt like she was making a statement about her worth.

The best book I have ever read on developing and sustaining intimacy in marriage is *A Lifelong Love Affair: Keeping Sexual Desire Alive in Your Relationship* by Joseph Nowinski.

In this chapter: I discussed how some sexual behavior is not about sex, how affairs arise from different reasons, and different results can be seen in your clients.

In the next chapter: I provide several examples of family dynamics your baffling client may have.

Chapter 23

Group Dynamics Affect
Your Client as a Couple
or Family Member

With your client before you, imagine standing beside them, all the groups that have a claim on them, and the dynamics that could be involved.

Thomas Fogarty's concepts
spell out family dynamics.

I have found Thomas Fogarty's concepts helpful in working with families. Below is a link to his collected papers: http://cflarchives.org/thomasfogartymdcollectedpapers.html

This article is one of his seminal articles: http://cflarchives.org/images/Triangles.pdf

Triangulation is one of the topics Thomas Fogarty discusses. As you listen to how your client relates to those around them, look for ways they may triangulate a third party to create a comfortable distance. The third party could be a person, a group of people, work, alcohol, or a hobby.

Arty explained that he had enjoyed having his own apartment for some years, making a good living working as an architect, and dating casually. Then, as he began to lose his hair and saw age thirty approaching, Arty felt like the oldest guy at the bar. He decided he needed to settle down. He had joined a Sunday school class at a large church nearby. There he met Lydia, who seemed like a perfect mate.

Now, after eight months of marriage, he felt like he was not very good at being married. Arty was an only child and had always been close to his parents. Lydia and his parents got along okay, but she insisted on cocooning herself and Arty away from his parents for the first months of the marriage. She said she wanted to feel like a couple rather than one part of an extended family.

Arty felt like Lydia was asking him to be emotionally intimate in a way the girls he had dated before didn't require of him. Luckily, he still had his golf buddies from college he could spend time with. Suddenly, golf became a preoccupation, and he played several times a week, much to Lydia's dismay. The arguments that followed led him to see me.

In treatment, he came to understand that he was using golf as a way to create a more comfortable distance between him and Lydia. I helped him reframe his difficulty with closeness as coming from a lack of practice rather than a sign that he was not meant to be married. Lydia accepted his early attempts, and they worked through this developmental phase of their marriage.

Family abuse dynamics can be surprising.

Much has been written about the dynamics of abuse. I want to mention one thing that surprised me because I believe it was not typical. People may relate to each other in ways that don't fit our preconceived notions of how things should be. In those instances, we can make errors because of confirmation bias.

For a thirteen-year-old, Ronnie dressed in a surprisingly bland style. I expected at least an outrageous saying on his T-shirt, since Ronnie was admitted to the psychiatric unit because his parents felt they could not control his behavior. It seemed curious that Ronnie was a model patient after admission, followed the rules, and got along well with the other patients and staff. After some time, he explained that he did not misbehave as a result of wanting to do something forbidden or an inability to control himself.

Ronnie saw misbehavior as a means to an end. He would misbehave provocatively. Exasperated over being unable to control him, Ronnie's mom would lose control and become violent toward him. Then she would become overcome with guilt at what she had said and done, embrace him, and tell him how much she loved him and how much he meant to her. She would promise that she would never do it again. Ronnie sought this intimate moment of closeness and love and was willing to do all the other behaviors to get it.

I would say that verbal abuse is the most common form of abuse and often goes unrecognized because it can be subtle. Suzette Hayden Elgin has written several books about recognizing and defending yourself from verbal abuse. Her first is called *The Gentle Art of Verbal Self-Defense*. She is a linguist, and the book teaches readers to recognize that when specific word structures are used, it is more likely to be verbal abuse. Elgin shows how people respond to the superficial content of the abuse without recognizing the abusive implications of how it is said. Then, she offers ways to counter the verbal abuse. For example, if someone says, "When are you ever going to take the trash out?" most people would devise an excuse rather than see the accusation of laziness, etc., that comes with the statement (Elgin 1985).

Because of how frequently therapists hear clients describe unrecognized verbal abuse, Dr. Elgin's book should be required reading.

Parent-child dynamics are fluid because all are continuously growing older.

A discussion of parenting dynamics is beyond the scope of this book. Nonetheless, I would like to make some observations from my own clinical experiences of how group dynamics can affect parent-child interaction.

As parents are raising their children, they and their children are continually growing older, making parenting more complex. When children become parents of their own children, they may appreciate their own parents more. Eventually, children may take on a more parental role in their parents' lives when parents grow older. Large families may make group dynamics even clearer as siblings take on different roles in response to family group phenomena.

As children grow and think for themselves, they may develop religious, political, or philosophical beliefs the parents find unacceptable. This development can generate guilt and conflict. Parents may feel they have failed if their child does not ascribe to their beliefs and may fear for their child's soul.

Some parent-child dynamics are not apparent at first. Clients have often complained about controlling mothers not providing enough freedom or respect. Initially, I believed the one-sided picture the client presented. Then I saw evidence that the client had attention deficit hyperactivity disorder and realized the mother was likely perpetually keeping her child from putting their hand into the fire and telling them to put down that fragile vase they were holding.

I once heard one mother described as controlling and overprotective. Later, I discovered she had lost a child and was willing to do anything to prevent that from happening again.

A teen might complain that their parents are like police officers. More history might reveal that the teen continually breaks house or community rules. In treatment, they are told they cannot expect their parents to stop acting like police officers until they stop acting like criminals. Change can begin when the teen finds the locus of control within themselves.

I heard complaints from adults who felt they had not been given direction and structure growing up because their parents were too permissive and not authoritarian enough. They said they were surprised that the world did not let them do what they wanted to do. They voiced dismay that parents had not helped them develop the resilience or self-control they needed to cope with adulthood.

If a child's birth altered a parent's hopes for their future, the child might sense they have the task of fulfilling that parent's unmet ambition.

Addicts may profoundly regret the effect their addictive behaviors have had on their family.

I want to mention a couple of things about how people suffering from addiction might feel about how their addiction has affected their families. What seems at first to be individually oriented behavior is later seen to be behavior driven by concern for the family group.

I was working in an alcohol inpatient unit when the Salvation Army brought in large bags of presents one December. In the Salvation Army's wisdom, they had not brought presents for the patients. Instead, they brought them for the patients' children. They knew how sad the patients were to not be able to get presents for their kids.

Regret is hard to bear.

On another occasion, a patient with an alcohol problem came into an inpatient facility after a suicide attempt. When I talked with him about his attempt, he explained that he was not tired of living, did not look forward to death, and was not depressed. He said he was just so tired of letting his family down and felt that if he were dead, he would not keep doing that to them. As he saw it, it would have been an altruistic suicide. He did not know how devastating suicide can be for a family.

Tackling a family problem from an angle may work better than the frontal approach.

Sometimes, clients have made progress, yet their families can't see it. The stories in this chapter all involve some sneakiness. Families come to therapy expecting the therapist to be all about change, and they don't like the therapist to rock the boat. The therapist can use their understanding of this dynamic to free the family from maladaptive patterns.

Juanita, a seventeen-year-old girl, was very responsible and had good social skills. She was ready to date, but her mom was worried about losing her closeness to her daughter. The family therapist working on my unit insisted that if Juanita were to date, she would have to come in at nine p.m. and tell her mom about the date. Juanita did precisely that. Then the therapist scolded her for not talking long enough with her mom and not giving more details. Mom was reassured that the therapist understood her. So the therapist assigned Juanita to go on another date and come in at ten p.m. Juanita was happy to have the extra hour. The therapist repeated the process with variations. Mom eventually realized she would not lose her daughter, and the therapist's insistence on the closeness was reassuring.

***

In this chapter: The families discussed in this chapter consciously met to care for each other.

In the next chapter: The group involved in the next chapter consciously met to work. Like the family, the workplace is awash with unconscious dynamics.

Chapter 24

Investigating How Your Client's Dynamics Play Out at Work

Both workers and bosses experience workplace stress that can come from a variety of sources and spark different dynamically driven behaviors.

Clients in management have dynamics influenced by workplace dynamics.

The workplace provides opportunities for your client's dynamics to emerge, including those around competition, failure, sharing, rivalry, favoritism, and mistreatment. If your client is in management, you may hear them complain about being unable to remove malcontent workers. They will feel stress from competing with local or international businesses. Keeping their sales numbers up and meeting payroll will be on their mind. They may discuss the rising cost of supplies, the supply chain's unreliability, and the shrinking profit margin. If they are in middle management, they might complain that they have the responsibility but not the power to carry it out. So they can't please their boss or their underlings.

Some job situations generate customers who demand immediate attention when things break down, like heaters, air conditioners, plumbing, or cars. Managers stress over being understaffed, losing profits, and having customers upset about waiting.

Managers often worry about motivating their employees. I have noticed that employees who excel in their roles usually get promoted into management positions, despite having little management training. They can feel like imposters but can't let on. You might occasionally hear about a secretary who is the brain behind her boss. Sometimes, that secretary is an adult child of an alcoholic who is good at covering for her boss and enabling him to get by. Workers who want to know something consult her and not the boss.

Your manager client may find that the pride older employees take in doing good work is not enough to motivate younger employees who grew up with a coaching model or prodding from a helicopter mom.

Managers and frontline employees worry about the future of the business. They can see business drop off and work hours cut. Employees are aware of the effects of creative destruction when someone else builds a better mousetrap, a cheaper item, or a more convenient way of doing something. Government employees can feel threatened by changes in policy and administration. Drug representatives' futures depend on how their companies' drugs are doing and whether some other company has a newer and better one.

Workplace group dynamics can subtly reinforce an employee's negative self-view

I worked for two companies that provided chart reviews to insurance companies to help them decide whether an insured continued to be disabled. My experience reviewing charts underscored what my clients had been telling me about how stressful workplace dynamics can be. By understanding your client's work situation, you can gain insight into their stress levels and more accurately assess the energy they have to devote to achieving their therapy goals.

Summer jobs in high school and part-time jobs in college may give people only a glimpse into what full-time work is like. Many clients are surprised by office power dynamics related to nepotism, sexual alliances, seniority, and blackmail. They were accustomed to being treated on their merit by teachers, who based grades on a test performance that could be measured. It was easy to believe a causal relationship existed between what they did and what happened next. It is difficult for them to understand the favoritism. It can trigger old resentments from having siblings favored over them. They are baffled by the injustice and lack of logic.

Here is how client dynamics may play out in the workplace when the client is new to the work group: When a new member joins a group, the group process typically involves assessing the new person's level of commitment to belonging. The group wants to know how much of themselves they are willing to sacrifice to be a member. Can they be the ones to get the coffee? Can they take the worst working schedule? Will they stay late or come in early? Some new employees don't understand that they are going through a group initiation. They see themselves as being discriminated against.

The initiation process and the favoritism are perceived as unfair. Employees may express their anger in passive-aggressive ways, such as not applying themselves, being late, or calling in sick. When you see them, they may have even had their boss call them down.

New employees are often judged based on their recent actions and the first impression they made. When I was in the U.S. Public Health Service, I saw service members who started out taking the same basic training. I would hear from one serviceman that he had graduated high in his basic training, gotten the advanced training he wanted, and was happy with his assignment and the service. Another service member, who did not do quite as well in boot camp, would have to wait for an advanced training placement and might not get his first choice even then. During the waiting period, he would become disenchanted with the service, act out somehow, and get assigned to a job he did not want in a place he did not want to be in. The service was a different experience for him than for the first guy, and it seemed to all follow from what happened in the very beginning.

If your client had problems with authority growing up, the work environment can provide a medium for acting it out.

Manual jobs require specific skills and can put workers under stress from having to work in a dangerous environment or sustain repetitive movement injuries. When you hear about a client working at one of these jobs, ask about injuries and chronic low-grade pain. If they are in law enforcement or firefighting, ask if they have lost coworkers.

I have often heard nurses say that hospitals count on their professionalism and fear of making mistakes that injure patients. Nurses believe that understaffed hospitals expect them to stay after their shift to complete paperwork they neglected while they were prioritizing patients' needs. Statistics vary, but it is safe to say that nurses can be adult children of alcoholics and accustomed to self-sacrifice; in this instance, it is the hospital and not their family that benefits. This practice is not true of all hospitals.

In some industries, it is a zero-sum game, and competition can make it feel like the company is a fight-or-flight group with an "us versus them" mentality. There is urgency. Productivity and creativity in beating the competition are valued. It is not a touchy-feely place, and laggards are left behind. When you hear about a client being in a pressure-cooker situation, ask about their blood pressure.

When doing a disability chart review, I noticed that I was reviewing the charts of several bank employees. I began to see how client dynamics were playing out with a bank merger in which a national bank had taken over a regional bank. The regional bank had been known for having a laid-back, welcoming atmosphere that treated customers like neighbors. They'd had employees who had worked for the bank for years and knew their customers. Their customers expected to be known. The national bank was more rigid and efficient, expecting regional bank employees to perform a lot of upselling. The regional employees felt their customers did not need and could not afford the upscale products. So, they did not sell many of them. Those employees would be warned and marginalized. The regional employees were stressed out by what felt like a toxic work environment. A crisis would leave them feeling overwhelmed with anxiety and missing work.

You may have a client who is stressed by a work secret. They may have seen someone in a compromising situation or discovered incompetence, cheating, abuse, rule-breaking, or deceit. Former soldiers have learned to take responsibility, follow standards of conduct, and sacrifice as part of a team, working together to accomplish a mission that is greater than themselves. They can be taken aback when they find themselves in a workforce that rewards loyalty and overlooks incompetence. Their competence makes them a target for sabotage by those who may be motivated to undermine them. When their excellence stands out, they can be mobbed by several coworkers who work together to undermine them.

Have you noticed that when you go out to eat, the server first apologizes? He has done nothing wrong and was not late. The server anticipates that you believe you should not be inconvenienced in the slightest way and are ready to complain. His belief is based on the experience of an increasingly demanding public that feels entitled. His job depends on tips and immediate customer satisfaction.

Is it any wonder that employees gather after work for a drink and a chance to commiserate? On those occasions, employees form alliances that employees who must go home to fulfill family obligations or get to a second job miss out on.

Other times, your client may be left out of an alliance based on a demographic they are not in. Being excluded may bring back a client's experience of dealing with cliques in high school or alliances in their family of origin. For the person who gets paranoid, it can be a trigger. They can't know what is happening if they are not there.

Remember the old saw, "Take a two-week vacation because if you only take one, they don't know you are gone, and if you take a three-week vacation, they have figured out how to replace you." Clients have told me that the resentment fellow employees felt at having to work harder in their absence led to mistreatment on their return. If work trauma was behind their absence, they would have to deal with this mistreatment as well as their PTSD.

Two excellent books come to mind: *Self-Sabotage Syndrome: Adult Children in the Workplace* by Janet G. Woititz and *The Bully at Work: What You Can Do to Stop the Hurt and Reclaim Your Dignity on the Job* by Gary Namie, PhD, and Ruth Namie, PhD.

After reading about these stressors, you might think people are uniformly relieved to retire. But sometimes, retirement comes prematurely, and people are not financially or emotionally prepared for the loss of role, purpose, and connections to others.

In this chapter: I gave a heads-up about workplace stressors and the possible dynamics that arise from them.

In the next chapter: I hint at how clients make mistakes related to cultural stereotypes.

Chapter 25

Culture May Underlie Baffling Dynamics

This chapter is about cultural dynamics.

**Seeing your client through the
eyes of your own culture may
blind you to their dynamics.**

We sometimes believe that, while we may not know
something about a person's background, we can make
assumptions about the nature of what we don't know. That is
especially risky when it comes to culture.

I'd like to share some surprises I encountered related to
culture.

When I was in the U.S. Public Health Service, Castro added
mental hospital patients to the boats leaving Cuba. I was
surprised that the paranoid patients claimed North American
science was controlling their minds. Their delusions were
culturally shaped.

On another occasion, I worked with American seamen who had traveled worldwide before they retired and came home to their wives, some of whom had never left the United States. These clients were fascinating because they had a meta-view of culture. A good culture motivates you to do what needs to be done. If your tribe relies on deer hunting for survival, it rewards you for hunting deer. The American seamen had transcended their culture, making it difficult for them to relate to their culture-bound wives. It also made it difficult for them to fit in. They felt most at home in the union hall, where they could swap stories with other sailors. You may see similar dynamics with returning service personnel.

Do not underestimate the role of shame in culture and how it might affect your client. Groups vary in how accepting they are of nonconformity. Sometimes, a member may have ideas that the group sees as heretical. A group may shame a member who has a child who is different and hold them responsible for the child being the way they are.

In this chapter: I gave a couple of examples of how culture affects dynamics.

In the next chapter: I will focus on parent-child dynamics.

Chapter 26
The Effect of Child-Rearing on Client Dynamics

A parent's self-doubt, drinking, overprotection, and rejection may have affected your client as a child. Your client recorded these experiences with their child's brain.

Your client's childhood brain recorded the information they share about their childhood.

When I hear about childhood experiences, I am wary of taking things at face value. These experiences were recorded with the mind of a child.

Children can be very concrete in their thinking. Once, I was in a park with a six-year-old who criticized me for crossing a paved path without looking both ways, like their teacher had taught them. There would never be a car or bicycle on that path, but the teacher's statement was seen as absolute.

The process of making and storing a memory is very complicated. Still, it is disassembled, with parts stored in different parts of the brain, then reassembled to be remembered. The memory of the overall meaning of past events, called the gist memory, is correct in general. But details might be incorrect. So the trauma memory might be legitimate, even though some elements are incorrectly remembered. I have come to rely on a client's gist memory, but I also realize that it was recorded as best as it could be by the six-year-old brain that recorded it.

I am told that the brain can repress memories at around age six. That is true in my experience because I mistakenly told a five-year-old I would take them for ice cream the next time I got paid and had to come through with the ice cream weeks later.

Children think other people's families do the same thing as theirs.

When your client tells you something strange their family does, consider that it might be true.

I was going through the cafeteria line at my college on a day when they were serving salmon croquettes. I asked for the syrup. The servers laughed at the idea that I would pour syrup on my croquettes. When I went home for Thanksgiving that year, I asked my dad about it. He told me he hated salmon, and my mom loved cooking salmon croquettes. He did not want to deprive her of the pleasure. So he killed the taste with syrup. My brother and I grew up thinking that was the way everyone ate salmon.

Parents often give their kids what they have, even though it may be meager by others' standards.

Clients frequently speak about poor parenting and abusive parents. Parents rarely have parent education. They grew up watching their parents and are influenced by that.

I recall a story about a young man who confided in his therapist about his father. He explained to the therapist that he grew up living next door to a rabbi. His father drank often and was absent from home. The young man spent many hours at the rabbi's house, where the kind rabbi was supportive and taught him many things about religion and life. One day, the young man was with his dad in a bar when his dad broke a beer bottle and held up the jagged edge. He told his son that he could use a broken bottle to protect himself in a fight. The young man asked the therapist what he thought. The therapist said, "Like the rabbi, your dad gave you what he had to give."

In the must-have book *Doing Psychotherapy: A Primer*, J. D. Gill, PhD, with brilliant clarity, covers the fundamentals of doing psychotherapy and offers profound insights into human nature. In it, she writes, "Life is about genuine connection and emotional truth. When parents fail, it is because of a problem with emotional truth, not because of a failure in discipline."

Clients may internalize their parents' self-doubts.

Another effect that child-rearing has on children is that the child internalizes a part of the parent. A client might feel terrible about themselves despite having loving parents.

Children watch their parents closely, emulate them, and internalize, or *introject*, what they see. That is, they identify with a parent's self-doubts and integrate that into who they are.

Parents may try to comfort their child by saying, "Don't feel bad about it. You're a Smith, and Smiths are just not good with math." It tells the child something is wrong with them but that it is okay.

Sometimes, a parent's self-doubt will show up as they continually fuss over a child's appearance or correct their behavior. It makes the child feel that being themselves is not good enough and that whatever they do is not good enough.

I try not to confuse this kind of criticism with my wife's remark as I go out the door, "Are you really going to wear that?" She just doesn't want me to look ridiculous.

I have had clients say that their mothers could not cope with their youthful beauty in the face of their own aging, so the mothers berated their children and tried to sabotage their romantic relationships.

The nationwide effect of wars, economic depressions, and pandemics may explain otherwise baffling client behaviors.

The effect of child-rearing on children is interwoven with the environment in which they are raised, and that includes political and economic events that affect the family. Clients from different generations have experienced historical events that shaped their behaviors. In the 1950s, there was a national polio epidemic. Parents whose children contracted polio felt guilty, like they had done something wrong and failed to protect their children. Several parents from that time became overprotective, and the children grew up feeling like the world was unsafe.

Have you ever been to an estate sale and had difficulty believing people could hold onto so much junk they no longer needed? Likely, those people grew up with parents who had experienced the Great Depression and were taught not to waste things for fear of needing them later. Sometimes, hoarding has a historical basis.

Clients may intentionally provoke rejection.

A child may seem oppositional when they feel rejected by their parents. By turning passive behavior into active, they provoke rejection. They now have an explanation for why they were rejected, as well as a sense of agency: They were rejected because they were bad. They tell themselves that they might not have been rejected if they had not been bad. It is less painful than thinking they would be rejected, even if they were good.

Adult children of alcoholics may have survived by not allowing themselves to feel, talk, or trust that others will come through.

Being raised in adversity can be a double-edged sword. Imagine having a parent who creates a situation that encourages a child to be self-reliant, care for their siblings, learn resilience by dealing with difficult situations, and push past their feelings to fulfill a compelling wish to make others whole. Would you believe it if I told you that parent has an alcohol use disorder? Now, go back and read the qualities I just described and ask yourself if those are not the qualities you see in many adult children of alcoholics. Adversity can sometimes build character, but it comes at a price.

The difference between a child who grows up in a more stable environment and one who grows up in a less stable environment is that the adult child of an alcoholic has to learn these skills to care for themselves, parent their siblings, and take responsibility because others don't. They have a profound desire to heal their parents, which sometimes translates into careers in the helping professions. Therapy may be harder for adult children of alcoholics because they need to notice their feelings, talk about them, and trust the therapeutic process.

When you notice your client worrying about and talking about everyone else in their life before they talk about themselves, ask yourself if they are an adult child of an alcoholic.

Lack of challenges may be disadvantageous.

I am not saying that it is good to grow up in an alcoholic family. On the other hand, the child who grows up in a home that's too centered on the child and has no challenges is less prepared.

If you help fretful, anxious parents deal with their anxiety, you will free up their kids to make mistakes and discover they aren't so fragile after all. You may explore the dynamics of this more by reading about the "good enough mother," a term coined by D. W. Winnicott, who, in 1953, wrote an article titled

"Transitional objects and transitional phenomena; a study of the first not-me possession" in *The International Journal of Psychoanalysis, 34,* 89–97.

This link from the Seleni Institute explains the concept. https://seleni.org/advice-support/2018/3/14/the-gift-of-the-good-enough-mother

---

In this chapter: I touched on how children change by taking responsibility, internalizing parental views, and recording events with a child's mind. Topics so far have dealt with gathering history, client resistance, client dynamics, factors in client-therapist interaction, and examples of different types of clients you might see. The following section will offer some ideas about doing therapy.

In the next chapter: I will discuss how to use Mike Rutherford's concepts about changing, homework assignments, positive reframing, careful wording, and indirect communication to promote progress.

Part 4

POINTERS ON DOING THERAPY

There is a passive quality about the first part of therapy in the sense that you are receiving information from the client and thinking about the data rather than decisively pursuing a particular course of treatment.

As you read further, you will notice a more assertive tone in how things are said, which parallels the therapist's shift toward being somewhat more active in the therapy.

As you know, when you make suggestions to clients and people in general, it is natural for them to resist being told what to do.

For the sake of brevity and clarity, I have chosen to become more direct, hoping my apparent pretentiousness will not discourage you from keeping an open mind about what you read. I trust you will continue to think of my recommendations as options, not imperatives, despite my use of the imperative voice.

Chapter 27

Having Mulled Things Over, Use These Tools to Act

Many techniques can cause change. Mike Rutherford's Equation for Change is explained as one scheme. Indirect communication, homework assignments, and the example you are setting are also tools.

Discover Mike Rutherford's Equation for Change.

You may have learned a specific set of techniques associated with the particular school of therapy that trained you. Having a foundation to build upon is an excellent thing. While I hope that this book increases your expertise in doing therapy, I will not advocate one school of therapy over another. Each offers valuable techniques. Instead, I would like to discuss what you might want to accomplish in therapy and how that affects the tools you use in your toolbox.

Employ Rutherford's equation to create a compelling vision and first steps toward change.

The history taken at the first visit acquainted you with the client. It likely suggested some ideas about what should be accomplished. Let us look at some treatment goals and valuable tools.

The heart of therapy is helping the client change. The first visit highlighted the client's dissatisfaction with the status quo. Now, it's time to help the client imagine how different circumstances can be.

The initial interview focused on finding out what was wrong.

You looked for signs and symptoms of things being wrong. The client revealed mistakes, shortcomings, deficits, and problems. Efforts were made to mitigate the negative content by reviewing the client's strengths and expressing your optimism that something can change.

On the second visit, reframe events positively. Stop asking why the client acted a certain way. Now ask them how they might create successful outcomes.

I am reminded of the behavioral shaping techniques experimenters used to get a bird to peck for seeds in the left direction. They ignore every movement the bird makes in the right direction, then drop grain each time the bird looks to the left. They shape the bird's behavior by reinforcing the desired behavior and ignoring the negative. S. G. Friedman, PhD, explains this in "Shaping New Behaviors" in *Good Bird Magazine*, reprinted on https://www.behaviorworks.org/files/articles/Shaping%20New%20Behaviors.pdf

In the first session, negative behaviors were identified; now, selectively reinforce the positive, hopeful behaviors and leave negative ones alone for now. In conversation with the client, your nod, smile, or short utterance, like "Yes" or "Uh-huh," is reinforcing. Look for early, not-yet-significant signs that something is better, then comment on it. Ask the client what they learned from the first session or what is different.

Reframe their wrongdoings as missing the mark in the process of getting better with practice. Focus on incremental change by dividing a long-term goal into a series of more manageable short-term goals. Help them develop a growth mindset and give up having to defend themselves as a static being.

When you hear of their shortcomings, your heartfelt acceptance, grace, and mercy model what you want them to experience toward themselves.

When a child feels known and loved by their parents, it makes it easier to accept that they are okay and frees them up to focus on caring for others as they have been cared for. They are also more comfortable recognizing their mistakes because they have a sense of being fundamentally okay.

This initial focus on the self in therapy could feel to the client like you are encouraging self-centeredness. But self-love is not selfishness. Being genuinely able to accept their own humanity frees them to become less self-conscious and connect with others. For those who were not so lucky as children, learning to accept their own humanity lovingly requires first focusing on self-understanding.

Identify factors amenable to change.

Look for and point out evidence of your client's value and resilience in the face of their situation. Encourage them to be curious about everyday life's more changeable elements. Where could they introduce some slight differences? Help them find a minor problem and develop a plan to change it. The idea is to show them that problems are not permanent.

Seek good circumstances in their current life to show them that, while some situations are bad, not everything in their life is going wrong.

They may think they have been singled out or are endlessly unlucky. While not minimizing how much their difficult circumstances have affected them, look for ways to normalize the parts of their situation they may have in common with others. For example, they did poorly on a difficult chemistry test, along with half their class. You might point out that they weren't the only student who did poorly while at the same time underscoring that you share their concern about passing the course.

Look for examples of how they have connected with others and help them identify when others have responded positively.

This article from *Positive Psychology* covers using positive therapy in more detail and offers active listening and exercise techniques: "How to Practice Active Listening:16 Examples and Techniques" https://positivepsychology.com/active-listening-techniques/

Like the Alcoholics Anonymous (AA) sponsor, your own example can be a vision of what change looks like for the client.

You can also use yourself as an example to help your client develop a compelling vision of change. Just as a child learns from watching their parents' behaviors, clients learn from observing yours.

Alcoholics Anonymous is a Twelve-Step program in which alcoholics meet anonymously to share their experience, strength, and hope to maintain their sobriety and live in recovery. In AA, alcoholics go to meetings where they see people in recovery and have regular contact with their sponsors, who are like mentors. They see how the sponsor can regulate their impulses and live in a way that makes their life manageable.

The alcoholic experiences the sponsor valuing them and sacrificing time and effort toward their well-being. When they relapse in their efforts toward sobriety, they experience the sponsor's mercy and forgiveness. The sponsor's tenacity in caring about them is a living statement of the belief that they, too, can recover. The sponsor's life embodies the inspiring vision of things being different.

When I think about AA sponsors, I am reminded of what Father Jim Finley said in an interview with Gary Moon of the

Martin Institute in discussing his book *Christian Meditation: Experiencing the Presence of God*:

> We are most powerless in being powerless to be anything else other than infinitely loved by God. That it is coming to the realization that nothing we do or say can make God love us more and nothing we do or say can make God love us less. The sole measure is the measureless expanse of Himself given to us whole and complete in and as who we simply are as precious in our brokenness (Moon 2016).

I have seen AA sponsors show that same redemptive love to the people they sponsor. That modeling and caring are also redemptive in therapy.

But the sponsor does more than care. They also set limits, boundaries, expectations, and norms. The same is true in therapy. Remember that therapy does not begin until acting out ends. Then, the client internalizes the conflict and feels the urge to start the change process. As I have mentioned, clients learn frustration tolerance by being frustrated and tolerating it in digestible, age-appropriate amounts.

Different therapists use different techniques to bring about change.

Next, in Mike Rutherford's equation for change, the first minor, successful steps are made. This is the how-to part. It is not enough to be dissatisfied and have hope; there needs to be a means to effect change.

Part of the how-to is helping the client examine what values they hold important. What do they see as the purpose of their life? Who and what have been important to them and have meaning? Reminding them of their core beliefs helps them build a base to make the first steps toward that interesting vision. They might draw on their spirituality and their parents' and mentors' teachings as sources of strength.

In the first step, you may educate and help the client build social skills. The client practices the new skills between sessions and returns to review how it went. These skills involve social learning and connecting with others as the client develops self-worth and confidence. You may teach mindfulness and affective containment techniques to help clients calm themselves. As the client undergoes trial and error, you respond with encouragement. Your support shows the client that failing is okay and part of the growth process.

Sometimes, you can carefully use humor to lighten the mood. For example, when a client tells me about a socially awkward moment, I might tell them how awkward I felt at a medical school prom in the early spring when I was wearing my cousin's hand-me-down white dinner jacket and everyone else was still wearing black tuxedoes. I then point out that both the client and I lived to tell our tales.

Another aspect of helping clients with the first steps is helping them get out of their own way.

Cognitive-behavioral therapy techniques help clients when they make mistakes in their thinking. It helps them make better decisions. And that can lead to changed behaviors.

Psychodynamic insight-oriented therapy uses techniques to help the client discover the unconscious conflicts that create resistance to change and paralyze their drive activity. You may help the client see how the repetition compulsion works to repeat past conflicts in their present life. They look for examples in the present of the most recent repetition.

These are just two of many therapies that help clients take those first steps. Suppose you have determined that a medical problem is also impairing their ability to take the first steps. In that case, you will want to do what you need to help them get medication to treat that impairment. If you believe your client has a borderline personality disorder, remember that dialectical behavior therapy (DBT) has been proven to help.

Do what you can to control
the treatment setting.

You may not have much control over the setting where you see your client. If possible, try to make it comfortable and warm. Your environment should reflect thoughtfulness, client consideration, and professionalism. You are trying to help your client feel emotionally safe.

Make some space between you and the client. Chairs should reflect equality. There should be privacy and quiet, but the client should know someone else is in the vicinity, like a symbolic monitor. A managed care company employee told me they looked at how old the magazines were in the waiting room to indicate quality care.

In treating trauma survivors, it is best not to wear cologne because the abuser might have worn that kind of cologne. It could trigger the client. Ask yourself if your clothing is appropriate. Evaluate the risks and benefits of wearing anything that shows your religious or political beliefs. Bumper stickers might also reveal something that puts off your client.

It is likely that some methods I am about to discuss do not fit your therapy situation. That's okay. Take what is helpful.

Choose your words carefully and consider asking clients to repeat what they have just been told.

I have had clients come up to my wife and me in a store and tell my wife how I had changed their lives by telling them to dye their hair cobalt blue and how it made all the difference. I could not imagine what they thought I had said because I knew I had not told them to dye their hair cobalt blue. The lesson is to be careful about what you say and what you put up in your office. Clients may misunderstand you.

If my wife tells me to get milk on the way home from work, I have no particular feeling about it. Then I forget the milk. My wife is mad. I have no milk for breakfast. The next time my wife tells me to get milk, I have some emotion attached to it. It has what is called a limbic valence. In therapy, the situation's urgency may lend some limbic valence to what the therapist says. However, I suspect it would surprise you to know that the client does not retain much of what you say.

If the client were a student listening to a lecture and not taking notes, you would not expect them to remember everything the lecturer said. The same is true in sessions. What if the lecturer prefaced their following remark with "This is going to be on the test"? Then your student is all ears.

So, there are times in your work with clients when you need to emphasize something important by repeating it or saying it in a way that lets the client know you believe it is important. If it is a direction related to a task, you might ask the client to repeat or write down what you just said. I've asked clients with attention deficit disorder or short-term memory difficulties to start a list of things they are going to need to remember to do after the session. Try not to overload your client's short-term memory, as I do now with yours.

While teaching has its place in therapy, therapy more often consists of the therapist fostering the client's efforts to do their own thinking about their situation with active listening, which might include occasionally restating elements of what the client just said in a way that clarifies it.

The client's conclusions are sometimes more memorable than those the therapist introduces. They have taken the time to stop, think, and absorb what has been discussed before reaching their conclusion. Their revelation may represent insight into what was previously an unconscious dynamic, and they may be freed up from having to repeat the pattern.

Sometimes, you do not have time to wait for the client to draw a conclusion or identify a pattern because the therapy is so abbreviated. It may be the last of only a few visits. In that case, you need to weigh the risk of their intellectualizing or denying what you told them against their never having a chance to hear the interpretation at all.

Using active listening and positive communication, carefully choose your words and reframe things to help your client imagine how things could be better and justify their hope. You remind them about their support system of friends, family, and faith. You identify times when they succeeded in working with others and using their self-discipline. Discuss available support groups and other resources for people who lack a support system.

As mentioned earlier, if you must confront a mistake they have made, try to sandwich the criticism between two positive remarks. For example, you might first say that you know what an effort they have made to be on time despite their busy schedule. They were late the last two times, but you feel like they will renew their efforts to be on time.

If you find yourself needing to set a limit on your client, it is helpful to explain your reasoning and how your expectation is a vote of confidence in their ability to tolerate the frustration of respecting it. Setting limits helps clients build ego strength as they practice patience, frustration tolerance, and waiting.

If you determine that your client is a visual learner, ask them if they get the picture. If they are an auditory learner, ask them if your words are clear as a bell. Match your vocabulary to their primary mode of learning whenever possible.

When you ask an oppositional client to do something they are reluctant to do, introduce an element of choice. Pretend you are trying to get your two-year-old child to put on their socks. Do they want to put it on the left or right foot first? Does your client want to start with 25 mg or 50 mg of medication, and how long do they want to try it before they raise the dose? There are two choices slanted in their favor.

You may not think a client knows your thoughts, but your body language can give you away. You may be unwittingly reinforcing something. When you are dealing with a potential abuse history, make sure you don't ask leading questions that suggest things to the client, and be careful with your body language.

Assigning homework can augment the treatment.

Sometimes, I have assigned homework tasks to clients. I may ask them to sit down with their parents or extended family members and review the family albums or pictures on their phones. I am trying to give them a way to be together and do something. But I also want to show them that they had some positive times together.

If I feel the client does not understand their parent's life or struggles, I will ask them to sit down with the parent and have the parent help them complete a structured life sketch. I show them that each line includes the date, the year of the parent's life, personal events, family life, health, and global events. They have a line for each year of the parent's life. Clients are often surprised by what they didn't know about their parents. This exercise can be an icebreaker.

Using indirect communication may reduce resistance.

If you need to confront a client, you might use indirect communication. For example, I may know from what I have read about a college student that they get drunk in the downtown bars every Thursday night. I pick a brief article on binge drinking as part of my reading selection that I ordinarily use to test their memory and reading comprehension. It seems to the client that I use it for all clients, but it indirectly conveys information and may be a conversation starter.

My gastroenterologist friend treated alcoholics with cirrhosis of the liver in a general hospital. Just before he discharged them to their family doctor, he would have the nurse come into their hospital room and adjust the blinds to darken the room. When he came in, he would visit them briefly. Then, as he walked just a bit away from their bed, he would say he was calling their family doctor. In hushed tones, just loud enough for the patient to hear, he would pretend to tell the family doctor how bad their lab studies were and what their prognosis would be if they didn't give up alcohol and get treatment for their alcoholism.

He had learned from his experience that patients listened more closely to what he was saying to someone else than they would if he put them in a position to defend themselves. He would later call the family doctor and say much the same thing.

Group therapy is beyond the scope of this book. If you want to learn more about groups, you might enjoy the chapter titled "Wilfred Bion's Theories about Groups" in *Search: A Guide to*

College and Life. I wrote this book with my wife (Roquemore 2020).

In this chapter: I discussed Mike Rutherford's concepts about change, ideas about reframing, homework ideas, and an example of indirect communication. Additional practical suggestions are scattered throughout the book.

In the next chapter: I address the importance of developing the habit of looking for the unexpected, the unusual, and clues in yourself about what is happening in therapy.

Chapter 28

Incorporate These Habits Into Your Treatment

Look for comorbid illness, developing diseases, and enzyme deficiency. Be sensitive when you correct or prompt clients. Understand how your position might intimidate clients, and pay attention to your own reactions.

**Your client may not be the only
one who is nonadherent at times.**

When I am tempted to lecture my clients about forgetting to take their medication, I try to remember what I am like as a dental patient. Then I think about how I rarely floss, miss brushing my teeth more often than I would like, and forget to put in my mouth guard.

How are *you* nonadherent to the treatment that has been recommended for you? Do you miss pills? Do you avoid sugar? Have you applied those creams as you should? It is a good habit to think about your own nonadherence. It will help you be less critical of your client, feel more merciful, and soften your approach when nudging them to do better. As mentioned earlier, think of two good things the client does and sandwich your criticism between them.

Knowing you will ask about
their self-care helps clients.

I went to Weight Watchers and attained my goal weight. The group support and the knowledge that I would be weighed affected my compliance. I got my lifetime pin but failed to grasp the "lifetime" concept. It turns out I needed accountability to keep my weight off.

My clients laugh at me when I explain that, in my training, I received a minor in nagging. They know that I, again, am about to remind them about the power of exercising, eating the right foods, and allowing themselves enough time to get adequate sleep. These things, which are thought to go without saying, should be said.

Incorporate the habit of asking:

- "How much sleep are you getting?"
- "What did you have for breakfast?"
- "What are you doing that is fun and gives you something to look forward to doing?"

You will not weigh your clients like Weight Watchers does, but asking about their health can make a difference. It is a concrete reminder that you care.

Do not underestimate how intimidating you might be.

It's good to remember that your status and persistence could be intimidating to your client.

I worried that the psychostimulants I was prescribing were raising my clients' blood pressure. So I bought a blood pressure cuff and took one client's blood pressure. It was dangerously high. I sent them directly to the emergency room. By the time they arrived, it had gone down to normal. They had what we call "white coat hypertension," which is named for a time when doctors uniformly wore white coats. The stress of being examined by a doctor and the uncertainty of what the doctor might discover had raised their blood pressure. After that incident, I stopped taking blood pressure in the office and asked my clients to get their blood pressure by using the machine at the local pharmacy.

Noticing your "tells" and your interaction with colleagues can help catch your mistakes.

By working with a team of colleagues, you can view how your client interacts with others.

Your observations may confirm or negate your assumptions about their dynamics and relationship patterns.

As long as confidentiality is maintained and you have the proper release, talking with colleagues about your clients can be helpful. Colleagues may see things you miss, which makes talking to them a good habit to incorporate into your practice.

When you are talking with your colleagues, notice if you tend to become sarcastic. It could be a clue that you are feeling helpless or frustrated with how the therapy is going. For example, is your frustrating client starting to feel like an opponent?

At such times, it might be helpful to remember the Serenity Prayer and consider what you have control over and what you don't. You may realize that you are just trying to do your best with the material the client presents. This realization may help you feel less tied to what the client, with their free will, chooses to do with your interventions.

Being sarcastic is just one of many tells you might notice. As a resident, my office was in a different building from my patients' inpatient hall. As I walked back to my office, I often noticed that I was singing a song in my mind. My supervisor suggested the song might reflect the unconscious process of the session, a background theme that went unrecognized. I am terrible at remembering lyrics, so I had to look them up. I was surprised that my mind often had accurately picked up on the process and somehow remembered lyrics I could not consciously recall. Notice what you are singing to yourself as a clue to what is going on in your mind.

Another tell might be your choosing a diagnosis for your client that is considered pejorative in popular parlance. My residency program wisely made Dr. Thomas Main's article "The Ailment" required reading for first-year residents. It shows how risky it can be for a patient to unwittingly frustrate the doctor's expectation that the patient will get well. https://bpspsychub.onlinelibrary.wiley.com/doi/abs/10.1111/j.2044-8341.1957.tb01193.x

Sometimes, a physical reaction can be a tell. I did medication checks at a residential treatment center for adolescents, some of whom were streetwise teenagers from urban centers. I found working with these clients almost uniformly made me uncontrollably sleepy. It was embarrassing to stifle yawns. Sometimes, you must make friends through idle conversation, but I could not find anything to say. I felt like I was a privileged white man who could not relate to their situations. Sometimes, they would smile when I brought up what I thought was a serious issue. Later, I realized their smile was nervous. They did not know what to say either. It felt like a stalemate.

Eventually, I had a meaningful conversation with a streetwise client who explained that he appreciated the kindness his house parents, teachers, and staff had shown him. He said he was tempted to let his guard down and own the sensitive parts of himself. Lamenting that it would be a mistake that he could not allow himself to make, he explained that if he did that, he would be a declawed cat thrown outside onto the street. He said it was sadistic to show him a different, better way, knowing he was going to have to go back to the streets.

He could not afford to engage with me in a conversation that might result in any fundamental change, so the superficial conversation that led to my sleepiness was self-protective.

I learned that supportive therapy makes more sense in some situations than others. I eventually realized I was sleepy when I felt helpless during a session. So, I watch for sleepiness. I also watch for feeling drained, which is another clue that I feel powerless.

Look for your client's
likely comorbid illnesses.

Incorporate the habit of thinking about comorbid illness. Sometimes, one disease leads to others in a domino effect. I see many patients who have diseases that are comorbid with depression, like heart disease. It is helpful to understand the connections because when you see one, you know to look for the other. Attacking the comorbid diseases can improve the depression outcome.

I have often seen some versions of this sequence of health events in my clients:

- Weight gain from a combination of lack of exercise and a diet high in carbohydrates and processed food leads to obesity. Obesity leads to metabolic syndrome (elevated blood pressure, elevated lipids, insulin resistance, and elevated weight) and silent inflammation.
- Silent inflammation fosters arthritis, headache, fatigue, and biome alterations, which contribute to intestinal problems. Arthritic changes in the back, combined with the stress of added weight, lead to chronic back pain and disc problems.
- Further obesity may lead to type II diabetes, knee problems, and sleep apnea. The elevated blood pressure, diabetes, and elevated lipids set the client up for heart disease and stroke.

In this cascade of illnesses, you can see several known contributors to depression that also complicate its recovery. A team approach that incorporates treatment for both mental and physical problems is more likely to be effective.

Recognize that disease diagnoses evolve.

Get into the habit of trying to expect the unexpected. You may encounter clients with unusual physical symptoms that don't fit into any known disease. Sometimes, the disease has yet to be clearly defined. Here is an example:

Some years ago, clients suffering from symptoms of what is now known as fibromyalgia complained to me that their doctors thought it was all in their heads. Eventually, doctors could understand some underlying mechanisms in fibromyalgia, which allowed them to determine which symptoms fit and exclude others from the confusing mix. Seeing that a new medication helped clients with a specific collection of symptoms further defined fibromyalgia.

Fibromyalgia clients were vindicated. What was first just a collection of seemingly random symptoms had finally evolved, in doctors' minds, into a legitimate disease.

Rare diseases may be overlooked, and some are termed "orphan diseases." Medicine is continually evolving, and new disease concepts are being discovered. Some diseases occur rarely; sometimes, you have clients with orphan diseases that are still poorly understood. Researchers are more likely to receive funding for research on illnesses that affect a large number of people.

Many clients have already googled their symptoms and have preconceived ideas about what is wrong with them. Sometimes, they are right. They may have an orphan disease or one that has not been identified yet. Their ideas should be considered, and their Google diagnosis may need to be evaluated. However, if you are a physician, be careful how you do the workup because spurious lab findings and test results can lead you down the wrong path, cost your client money, and offer false hope.

If you are working with a client's physician, it can feel awkward to broach the subject of the client's unusual symptoms. You might worry that the doctor will wonder if you are being gullible and bothering them for no reason.

Seasoned therapists will tell you that you will be better received if you do some background reading, present your case concisely and logically to save the doctor's time, and show your reasoning.

It's okay to risk looking foolish. You are being an advocate for the client's well-being. You may be surprised when the doctor is grateful that you pointed out something that was not obvious.

Consider using the tiger story as a crude predictor of enzyme deficiency.

When a client tells me that they and others in their family scrupulously avoid anxiety-inducing situations, I suspect that they may have an inherited difficulty in methylating folate, which leads them to take longer to calm down. I tell them my tiger story to get an idea of how they and their family handle an anxiety-producing situation.

First, I should warn you that my tiger story has not been tested or proven to be reliable or truly predictive, but I have found the results sometimes useful as an additional clue. Using the tiger story might be a helpful habit to develop.

I ask them to imagine they are standing on a field. Next to them are their parents, siblings, and me. I tell them I have a completely normal body in this situation. We all see a tiger coming at us from two hundred yards away. We all have a fight-or-flight reflex, which can lead to anxiety. We sweat, our hearts beat faster, and we get ready to run or fight. Then we simultaneously realize that it is not a tiger. It is a big dog, and dogs don't scare us. Everyone begins to calm down. I calm down at a normal rate. I ask the client how fast they calm down by comparison. Does it take them the same time, twice as long, or somewhere in between? What about each member of their family?

I may also tell them my highway patrol story.

I ask them to imagine they are on a superhighway driving 60 mph in a 60-mph zone. They see blue lights in their rearview mirror and realize that a highway patrol car is approaching them fast. They wonder if they will be pulled over. Then the patrol car goes by them and pulls over someone else who was farther down the road. I ask them how long it takes to calm down after they realize that the patrol car wasn't after them.

If the client describes a pattern of themselves and one parent or a sibling taking longer to calm down, I order a genetic test. I am looking to see if they have problems methylating folate because they lack enough methylenetetrahydrofolate reductase enzyme. I am surprised at how many people have this.

It may take weeks or months to see the full effect of taking L-methylfolate, but clients tell me it makes such a difference. They are not as fearful of going into social situations. They don't dread being a little anxious because they know they can calm down. To learn more about this, go to this link: https://genesight.com/genetic-insights/understanding-the-mthfr-gene-mutation/

Another clue that they may have a problem methylating folate is if they are given Adderall for their ADHD and become excessively anxious.

In this chapter: I illustrated the three C's—Caring, Competence, and Carefulness—which were mentioned in the introduction. Caring was demonstrated by sandwiching criticism between two positives and asking about a client's wellness activities. Competence included identifying tells and refocusing on the task of therapy. Carefulness was shown in not overlooking comorbid illnesses and enzyme deficits.

In the next chapter: I examine how clients are stressed by having to lead, quit a job or relationship, try new behaviors, or experience failure.

Chapter 29
Identify Clients'
Stressors to Treat Them

Making decisions is risky and stressful, whether it is choosing the correct life path, leaving a partner, accepting the role of leader, or trying out a new behavior. You may be standing beside your client at a crossroads in their life.

Clients may struggle to quit when they should.

We live in a society that expects people to play through the fourth quarter of the football game with an injury. "No pain, no gain." When I tell clients that knowing when to quit is a life skill and that quitting should be a consideration, they look at me like I am un-American.

Quitting can be a sign of self-esteem. Quitting says, "I am not putting up with this because I deserve better." It takes some self-confidence to quit, knowing change is needed. The quitter has recognized and acknowledged that they have made a miscalculation. James Baldwin said, "The meaning of revelation is that it must be borne."

When discussing the pros and cons of quitting with your clients, keep in mind that it may require planning before they can take the plunge. Quitting may affect multiple people in their support system. When a client quits their job, it affects their coworkers, who may now be short staffed, and their family, who may suffer financial stress.

While weighing the pros and cons, your client may find that certain actions can help regardless of their decision. You might encourage them to use the time to get more education, become more fit, or acquire more job skills.

Some clients mourn the path not taken.

Identifying a client stressor may be more difficult when the stressor is hidden among good things. Having children or choosing a college, a mate, a city, a job, or a house all require saying no to other options. Many choices are mutually exclusive. Saying yes to one thing may mean saying no to all others. You can't always have your cake and eat it too. Loss may be inherent in choice.

You may view a client celebrating a joyous event and find they are unexpectedly sad. For example, a job promotion may mean the person must leave their coworkers.

When people are middle-aged, they have already made choices that sent them down different paths. Some bells they have rung cannot be unrung. Perhaps they spent years getting themselves out of the holes the poor decisions dug in their youth. They wonder why they have continually picked rocky road when there were thirty-five other flavors.

Part of your work with middle-aged clients may involve helping them make peace with their choices and see how to make better ones in the future. It may start with helping them grieve.

The persecutory superego, which is made up of a collection of negative self-concepts clients internalized as children, is as relentless, as it is unforgiving in its unrealistic expectation of perfection. It demands, "Prove yourself!"

I mentioned earlier that you never know whether you are a small light in someone's great darkness. Maybe that darkness is a severe depression. But sometimes, it is created by a client's harsh, persecutory superego. It is dangerous because, on the surface, you see a client who is successful and very likable, with a loving family and every reason to like themselves. The stressor you need to identify is not visible.

You don't know what their parents told them that has been incorporated into their superego. Those comments could be very damaging. They may have had to meet unrealistic expectations to get parental approval. They can't relinquish their childhood belief in their omnipotence, which leads them to expect perfection from themselves.

With childhood's concrete thinking, they may have incorrectly incorporated religious and cultural teachings, which they see as judging them harshly. It may have never occurred to them that Heaven might not have a gate to keep people out and that their whole life does not have to be about proving they deserve to be inside.

They may have concluded they *were* a mistake instead of someone who *makes* mistakes. They may have absorbed a bullying parent's statements about their self-worth.

You may lose your job and believe you can eventually find another. But your client may berate themselves, remind themselves that their parent was right about them being a failure and feel life is not worth living. The same stimulus elicits different responses, depending on what the client tells themselves. You need to discover what the client tells themselves rather than assuming they think like you. You are looking at their obvious strengths; they are looking at their failings compared with their unrealistic standards.

Some clients feel you are a paid cheerleader and discount any direct reassurance you might give. If you expect that response, you might show them the illogic of their mistakenly incorporated superego harshness.

You may think the self-discovery process in therapy will result in your client having greater self-esteem. They may fear that they will discover they are as bad as they have been told they are.

Your client may deal with their failings and harsh superego by putting their conflict into behaviors and acting it out. Be aware that if their situation changes and they can no longer act out, they may have to internalize the conflict, which may result in depression. This process sometimes happens to people who are imprisoned or become physically disabled.

Good people may make bad choices when they feel desperate.

You may not know how desperate your client feels about their situation. They may be alone and feel unbearably lonely. They need to feed their family. They sense that their safety and the safety of their family are threatened.

You may not suspect that they have done something wrong because they present as an honest rule follower. Their behavior seems puzzling when their stressor is not apparent, like there is a secret you don't know. They may not talk about it for fear of compromising someone else. Consider discussing what you think are analogous situations to convey the notion of grace and acceptance without revealing the secret.

For example, when I was first in private practice in my early thirties, several clients told me they had paid me in cash, but there was no record of their payments. So they were rebilled for the same appointment. After this happened multiple times, I realized that my secretary, an ordinarily conscientious and efficient worker, was embezzling funds.

I did not confront her about embezzling. As an excuse for firing her, I instead talked about how she had not allowed clients to reach me when they needed to. I felt betrayed, but we were in a tiny town. I was worried she would stir up trouble if she became very disgruntled over her firing.

She was the major breadwinner in her family, and her pay may not have been enough to make ends meet. That does not justify her behavior, but it suggests that she could have been a good person in a possibly desperate situation.

I was so surprised and felt stupid for not catching her sooner. I did not wait long enough to think it through. Today, I wonder whether a frank discussion might have resulted in her working out a way to pay me back and keep her job. My reluctance to confront her gave her no chance at redemption. I am not trying to give administrative advice, but if your secretary never takes a day off, be suspicious and remember that good people may have done regrettable things when they felt desperate. Embezzlers don't want you looking at the books while they are on vacation.

Clients may overcorrect
when trying new behaviors.

This case illustrates how a client may go overboard when they try new behaviors.

Mary Katherine looked like something the cat had dragged in as she slumped in her seat and apologized for being late again. I told her that some clients who also have attention deficit disorder use calendars and phone alarms to help them organize their days and get their assignments in on time.

At our next appointment, Mary Catherine arrived promptly and was excited to show me her schedule book with colored tabs and detailed appointment lists. Her smartphone now had multiple alarms. On her new bulletin board, she had placed different assignments by date with different-colored sticky notes by subject. She lamented that she had spent so much time getting organized that she had not had time to study for her test. In trying a new behavior, she had overcorrected.

I have a favorite story about power steering that I use to illustrate initial overcorrection. My example, however, also demonstrates the need for therapists to update examples when talking to clients of different ages.

There was a time when cars all had manual steering. Then, power steering, which was very responsive to slight movement, came along. When people started using power steering, they would turn the steering wheel to the right, and the car would go far to the right. Then, they would turn the steering wheel to the left, and the car would veer far to the left. They overcorrected in both directions until they got a feel for power steering. Hearing my old-fashioned example, some students found themselves trying hard not to laugh at me and missed the gist of the analogy.

Being the alpha dog may be a stressful responsibility for you and your clients.

When you are told that someone is the alpha dog, you may assume that the person has fought off all the competition and is the fiercest. But being tough is only one aspect of being an alpha dog.

In our family, my furry Bichon Frisé, Sophie, believes she is the alpha dog. She assumes the stalking position, ready to fight, when she approaches strangers walking their dogs. Sophie accepts this responsibility to protect her pack—my daughter, my wife, and me. She barks at people walking past our house to protect us and let them know she is to be reckoned with. She takes her role seriously, but she's a nervous wreck, running from door to door and barking at them.

Alpha dogs lick their pack members to keep them clean. Sophie is businesslike as she systematically licks my face from ear to ear every time I lie down on the floor to do exercises.

I tell this story to help you understand what your clients who are chief executive officers (CEO), business owners, or managers feel about protecting their pack. They feel that it's not just what they do, but who they are. This feeling creates pressure when employees risk losing jobs, business decisions unintentionally hurt people, or employees struggle.

Being a pack leader is just one part of a CEO's complex job. Bombarded by problems all day, they can come home desensitized. You may hear their partners complain that after a day of handling enormous problems, their spouse seems unmoved by their struggles, which don't seem serious enough to register.

Helping executives cope with the effects their position has on them and others does not mean they have to relinquish their leadership role; however, recognizing the unique stressors they face can be beneficial.

You may not realize it, but your position and how clients see you might lead you to feel some of the responsibilities of an alpha dog. You may not recognize how much stress your position places you in or how you are becoming desensitized to it until you are temporarily removed from it.

I did not appreciate this stress enough until I took a Globus tour of Europe. It was clear that the tour guide was the alpha dog. He knew details of European history, anticipated all our needs, guided us through any difficulty, and told us what to do as needed. I loved it. Having temporarily taken off the mantle of clinical responsibility, I wasn't the alpha dog. The experience made me realize how people can long for an authoritarian leader. But at the end of the tour, I felt abandoned and was waiting to be told where and when to go to the bathroom.

Being a therapist is challenging but worth the effort. Your life is richer for it. Like the CEO, you feel needed and purposeful.

Your clients may have trouble leaving their character-disordered partners.

One feature of character disorders is that the person experiences their maladaptive behaviors as ego-syntonic. That is, they see their behavior as just part of who they are. They don't have a problem. They are usually not worried enough to want to see you. They don't have a stressor. They *are* the stressor.

Your client may be worried about a boyfriend or girlfriend who is engaged in maladaptive behaviors. To avoid cumbersome language, let's make the girlfriend a client who is concerned about her character-disordered boyfriend.

The girlfriend experienced the boyfriend's indifference as alluring and a challenge to be good enough to gain his attention. Later, she will complain about him being insensitive and self-centered. Initially, she is attracted by his devil-may-care, fun orientation. But later, she will say he is impulsive and makes poor decisions. His spontaneity attracted her, but later, she will complain about his lack of planning and direction.

Because he did not like to think about problems, she made the hard decisions and enjoyed being in control. His mother told her she was the best thing that had ever happened to her son. Later, she realized his mother was tired of cleaning up her son's messes and was excited about passing the torch to her.

Your client initially prided herself on seeing the good in her boyfriend. Later, she wondered why she could be so blind to all his faults. The odd thing about him is that he was not actively evil or persistently hurtful. He was not actively doing anything. He was just thoroughly disappointing.

Eventually, he finds her less attractive because she feels like a mother to him. She loses interest because he doesn't feel like a man, but more like a son. Finally, he is particularly disappointing to her when he moves on to greener pastures like a parasite that recognizes the host is not doing well.

Even though she wants him to make significant changes, he takes the path of least resistance and picks someone else.

Your job as the girlfriend's therapist is first to make an educated guess about what kind of character pathology this boyfriend has. (Without seeing the boyfriend in person, a diagnosis cannot be made.) There may be mixtures of narcissistic, borderline, sociopathic, immature, and inadequate features. Determine if the boyfriend is a malignant narcissist. Some narcissists are dangerous to leave.

Some girlfriends don't like to see themselves as giving up, being disloyal, or being a poor mate selector. Some have trouble realizing the magnitude of their mistake.

Clients may provoke the
behaviors they expect to see.

Some clients' behavior is the source of stress you are trying to identify. Standing in a long line at the cosmetics counter of a department store, I listened to a clerk curtly answer a demanding customer's questions. After the customer left, the next customer approached the clerk with a smile, and the clerk treated them warmly and courteously. Each customer would have drawn different conclusions about the clerk. If you were treating the demanding customer, they would paint the clerk as curt. They expected the clerk to be difficult and provoked that behavior by being demanding and accusatory.

As you hear a client describe others, consider that their behavior may bring out the worst or best in others. Their description may not accurately reflect how others are at other times. This could give you a distorted picture and set you up to draw the wrong conclusions about your client's environment and relationships. They may be sabotaging themselves without realizing it.

In a hospital nursery, you might be impressed by how different the apparent temperaments of various babies are. Some coo and others seem fussy and cry.

Just like you might find some babies almost irresistible to pick up, there are people in the adult world who seem more approachable than others. These approachable people are the ones you walk up to in Walmart to ask where the batteries are. They tell you they are not employees and that they get that all the time. They have high approachability.

As you listen to clients talk about how others treat them and their conclusions about humanity, wonder how their temperament might affect others' interest in approaching them.

Your expectations about your client can also shape your client's behavior.

I worked in a hospital for dual-diagnosed adolescents when insurance allowed them to stay long enough for their work in therapy to help them make changes in their character. The therapeutic community used a level system that incrementally rewarded progress with more freedom and responsibility.

Each week, we held a community-level meeting to discuss and adjust each client's level based on their behavior that week. Seeing how the same client acted differently with different staff members was fascinating. That led to differing opinions among staff members about a particular client's level. Some staff were looking for the pathology in the client's behavior, and others were more focused on looking for progress. It seemed like each saw what they were looking for, and the clients seemed to respond to their expectations. I was reminded of the power of confirmation bias and the self-fulfilling prophecy.

In this chapter: I discussed how clients may create stress by provoking behaviors in others they dread or continually feeling they need to prove themselves. I reminded you that real-life stressors are involved in making important decisions about changing relationships, taking on responsibility for leading others, and doing something new. These situations are not as uncommon as the ones you will encounter in the next chapter.

In the next chapter: You may find yourself outside your comfort zone when your lifestyle has little in common with your clients'. Or maybe you simply don't like your client. Perhaps you have been asked a favor you find questionable or received a gift. I suggest that you remember your guidelines, making peace with yourself and trying to abide in the situation as you allow it to unfold, then suggest a path forward.

Chapter 30

Anticipate These Various Awkward Situations

It would not be unusual to encounter unlikable clients, clients who request support animals, show maladaptive behaviors, offer gifts, and are reluctant to talk. You could also have deprived clients and wealthy clients. If you can anticipate these potentially awkward situations and approach them with thoughtfulness and flexibility, you may have a better outcome.

Provide the same treatment to your unlikable clients that you provide to others.

Everyone encounters people who, for some reason, just rub them the wrong way. I had a client I could not bring myself to like. She seemed disagreeable, opinionated, and spiteful. Her appearance and manner reminded me of an abrasive person from my past who had said hurtful things to my best friend, which made me angry.

While I tried to hide my feelings and thought I was treating her like any other client, I expected her to see through me and have that influence the outcome of the treatment. To avoid the anxiety of being consciously aware of my angry feelings, I did precisely the opposite of what I felt: I used the defense mechanism of reaction formation. I was overly careful to act professionally despite not wanting to treat the client. I was excessively conscientious. I made a point of listening carefully and offering encouraging comments. I made sure the treatment plan was appropriate and followed the protocols. I scheduled her as frequently as I would any similar client. It shocked me when, over time, she got substantially better. Because the treatment was essentially appropriate, it worked, despite the reaction formation that led me to overdo it somewhat.

My wife and I went on a cruise, which included a trip to a maple syrup factory in Canada. I bit into a maple syrup lollipop, and the veneer on my front tooth came off. Until I could see a dentist, I made do by wearing my night guard during the day. Looking in the mirror, I saw the face of the woman I had not liked. The night guard had given me a "resting bitch face." If I had passed myself on the street, I would have thought I was a disagreeable character. I wondered how many other people are misunderstood in the same way. I'd misjudged my client because of the negative connotations I had attributed to her appearance and manner.

You cannot always control who you treat. Applying what you know about treatment and going by the guidelines can help you when your heart is not in it. Sometimes, you must remind yourself that you're a professional and do the best for the patient, even if you would rather be anywhere else.

Avoid providing support animal certifications that could compromise a career.

When asked to complete a certificate for an emotional support animal, please weigh the benefits against the risks to a client's future career. If a job requires a security clearance, an employer may request records. If the applicant objects, this might be disqualifying.

That a client has, at some point, needed an emotional support animal may suggest to an employer that the client lacks the self-confidence or resilience the job requires. Employers may not be excited about having to make accommodations for an animal in the workplace.

Point out disparities as a way of confronting maladaptive behaviors.

Another awkward situation comes up when you must confront your client's maladaptive behaviors. In your client's eyes, you may flip from being an empathetic rescuer to what some kids would call a "mean mommy" who says no. While the quality of your relationship is a significant factor in the effectiveness of therapy, you may need to incur your client's displeasure with you to help their recovery.

One way to address the maladaptive behavior is to highlight the discrepancy between their stated intentions and their actual actions. For example, you might say, "You have talked about wanting to be more sociable, but I see you are wearing a T-shirt that says, 'I'm late because I didn't want to come.' How does that work toward your goals?"

You may find yourself having to confront a client's dangerous behaviors. For example, clients may want to drink while taking medications when that is not recommended. Cognitively or visually impaired clients might insist they can still drive. You may need to educate your client more in these instances. You could point out how your client's wish for health contrasts with their wanting to engage in dangerous behavior.

Patient gifts require different, nuanced responses.

A client giving a therapist a gift is just one more client behavior that is grist for the therapy mill. It may seem impolite and ungrateful to ask a client questions about their gift-giving. Here are some guidelines to consider when you find yourself in the awkward situation of being given a gift:

- If the item is expensive, most therapists would not accept it but would thank the client for their thoughtfulness. You can remind them of the professional nature of your relationship. You do that delicately and warmly. You might also consider whether not accepting the gift is a grave insult in your client's culture.
- If the client is a child who has made something for you, accept it to avoid crushing them by rejecting something they made. They may not understand the rationale behind your rejection.

One client, when asked about a gift she had created herself, told me she was not sure I would remember her after our sessions stopped. She hoped the present would help me remember. When I see her gift, I wish she had recognized how exceptionally kind she was and how worthy she was of being remembered, regardless of whether I had a gift.

I still have a small box a girl made in her art therapy at the hospital where I was treating her for her schizophrenic illness. She had a very oppositional relationship with her dad and repeated that relationship with me. Her gift had multiple meanings. It was a peace offering, a kind of undoing of her anger toward me, and a way of nonverbally telling me she appreciated my hanging in there. It was also a way of asking me not to desert her despite her behavior. Rejecting the gift would have felt like I was rejecting her.

An older client, who was somewhat paranoid, often baked bread. She would bring me one of the loaves when she came for her medication checks. Later, I realized she feared me and that the bread was meant to appease me. I should have suspected her ambivalence because the bread frequently had some burned edges. She was giving me a mixed message.

Abiding with clients is a skill gained through practice.

Some situations are dire. You will treat people who are dying. Your clients may have miserable life situations beyond anyone's control. You may feel helpless and uncomfortable when you're unable to make a direct impact. Don't discount how important it is to just be with the client, even if you can't do something to change their situation. Sometimes, a client's relatives, who love them very much, feel overwhelmed by the client's intense emotions. You might have enough distance to do what they want to but can't.

I had an odd introduction to the power of just being with a client when I was a first-year psychiatric resident. I was working with a young woman who had stopped talking before her admission. Based on her history, the staff hypothesized she was mute because she was afraid of what she would do or say and was paralyzed by that fear.

Previously, in the 1970s, we used cold, wet sheet packs to help agitated clients regain control. A client would lie down on a kind of bed and be wrapped in sheets so they could not move but could breathe easily and be comfortable. Because their body would heat up from being wrapped up, the sheets would be wet with water. (One of our residents thought it was barbaric and asked to try it. She told us it was rather pleasant and that she had felt warmly held. Sometimes, clients acted out to get wrapped up. I suppose this was the forerunner of the weighted blanket or the thunder blanket used for dogs afraid of lightning.)

So, my client would be wrapped up for our therapy session day after day. I would come in, sit beside the bed, and simply be with her. Sometimes, I would talk about nothing in particular. But mostly, I would sit beside the bed. The idea was that by being unable to act on her impulses, she would talk about them. Days went by, and I felt like I was not getting anywhere. My staff was still supportive of the idea. At some point, I found peace in being with her in silence. It felt like a kind of "oneness" when we joined in a common silence. When I could accept that she was not talking and she saw that I continued to come, it began to have an effect. One day, she looked at a brown bag I had with me and said, "What's in the bag?" I explained that my lunch was inside. That was the beginning of her talking, and she made progress after that based in part on the foundation of our shared silence.

Realize that you cannot make taking out the trash fun.

Some things, like taking out the trash, are just not fun and never will be. People don't want to do them. When they do, it may be because they view the task as a means to a later reward that outweighs the aggravation. When your client appears unmotivated, you may be chasing your tail when you look for some hidden dynamic. Maybe the nature of the task is the problem.

People have different degrees of frustration tolerance and ability to delay gratification. If a client is too depressed to do something, an antidepressant might help them feel motivated, but it will not make the trash fun to take out.

I was working with a client who said he did not want to do anything. I looked at his ambivalence, his difficulty enjoying things, and aspects of his depression, only to find out that he had a different reason for being stuck. He believed he had to do all the chores before doing anything fun. He couldn't get himself to do the chores, so he never got to do anything fun. I can hear his mother yelling, "You can't go out until you have cleaned your room!"

Deprivation can lead to entitlement. First, focus on what leads to deprivation.

One drawback of being deprived is that it leads to a wish for compensation. When I have had to put up with an exasperating software program, I feel entitled to break my diet and eat the remaining large piece of peach cobbler before anyone else can.

If I were your client and told you this, you might point out why I should not eat the cobbler. You might work on my impulse control issues or my narcissistic feelings of entitlement that make me believe the rules don't apply to me.

Instead, consider working on what led to my sense of deprivation. If I improved my software skills or upgraded my software, I might not feel deprived. Ask if I am failing to do nurturing and rewarding things elsewhere in my life. Helping me focus on the positives might make software-related deprivation less critical.

Sometimes, it's not seeking compensation for being deprived that drives our behavior. It is that enjoyable things are, well, enjoyable.

Having wealth can be emotionally stressful.

I have talked about my sweet dog, Sophie, and how protective she is of us. All our neighbors would confirm our belief that she is an exceptionally loving dog. That is, until you give her a bone. She grabs it quickly and takes it to a safe place. She won't go to bed. Instead, she stays up to guard her bone. When we approach her, she growls. If we get too close, she may bite.

When I think of how obsessed Sophie is with having a bone, I think about some of my affluent clients who fear losing what they have. There is nothing wrong with having things. Yet, because they have something, they feel like everyone wants to take advantage of them or has a hidden agenda. Therefore, they police themselves by looking for those who don't belong in their group. Rather than being inclusive, it is an exclusive group of wealthy people. The problem with belonging to an exclusive group is that you might be excluded if you have a blemish, like a mental illness or, as was the case in the television series *The Gilded Age*, are divorced. I am grateful to clients who will see me because I know some of them risk being labeled blemished.

Sometimes, what looks like a symptom is not.

Remember that a symptom that looks like mental pathology may be explained by a lack of health education or some other nonmental health reason.

I remember a fellow who told me that when he was in the living room where his wife died, he heard soft voices. He did not seem to have any other symptoms of psychosis, and he wasn't having alcoholic hallucinosis. The source of the sounds came from a Christmas ornament whose battery was almost dead, so the tune it played was too soft for him to hear at first.

Considering brain networks can give you more insight into how your baffling client thinks.

Understanding how the brain works can help you better understand unusual client situations. Below is a comprehensive video overview from Visceral.Labs69-wo7su: *The Four Main Brain Networks (Salience, Default Mode,*

Central Executive, Task Positive) https://www.youtube.com/watch?v=cfwQDS8r80s

---

275

In this chapter: I discussed situations that require seeing things from a client's unusual perspective and collaborating in the treatment while being guided by what you have been taught.

In the next chapter: I will discuss some obstacles to treatment. These include your clients' lack of psychological mindedness, fear of stigma, and distorted views of you.

Chapter 31

Notice Obstacles in the Treatment of Baffling Clients

It might be a mistake to assume clients see therapy like you do. Differences lead to delays in treatment, erratic or surprising progress, and possibly the need to set limits.

Clients differ in when they need treatment.

My patient was a frail woman in her late sixties who was frightened to be in a big hospital in a big city far from her farm. Her chart noted that she had been having auditory hallucinations and frequently talked to the trees. I asked her husband how long it had been going on. He told me she had been talking to the trees for four years. I asked him what led him to bring her in for treatment. He said that she had stopped cooking a week earlier.

That was a lesson in how what is clinical to one person is not to another. You may hear your client tell you about a horrible situation, such as domestic abuse, and assume they would not have tolerated it for long. Clients may be embarrassed to tell you how long it has been happening.

Adults may take longer to notice children with attention deficit disorder without hyperactivity than they would children with hyperactivity. Children without the hyperactivity can stay in their chairs and not aggravate teachers or parents. Their inattentiveness can be dismissed as laziness or a lack of motivation. They are no trouble. If they are doing well in school, no one notices that they must study twice as hard.

Fear and stigma can delay treatment.

When I was a kid, I was afraid of what the doctor would do to me. Now I fear what he will tell me is wrong. Clients may delay treatment when they fear what they may discover. They may delay because of costs or because they don't understand the significance of their symptoms. Sometimes, they delay because they're in denial or want to avoid stigma.

I have seen clients whose parents had mental illnesses that were improperly treated. The children delayed seeking treatment because they were skeptical about what a profession that failed their parents could do for them.

As I have mentioned, different cultures may regard seeking treatment as a sign of a lack of religious faith.

Misinformation can be an obstacle in treatment. In 1982, I had a client in a rural area who had to lock herself in her home's bathroom to avoid her neighbors trying to perform an exorcism to remove a demon. The neighbors believed she had a demon as a result of seeing a psychiatrist. They had bought into the idea that educated people are not God-fearing and that the secret nature of our meetings hid a kind of brainwashing with sinful intent.

My wife and I allowed the neighbors' church to baptize members in our creek. But when we moved away, one of those neighbors told my wife, "We don't need your kind around here."

The rooster on our farm had a bad habit of getting into my neighbor's henhouse. She would call me and insist that I come and get him. Unfortunately, he was too fast for me to catch during the daytime, so I had to wait until he roosted at night. I can't help but think that part of our outcast status was due to her still being upset about our rooster getting into her henhouse.

Clients dump revelations on their way out the door.

Time limitations can impede treatment. Before letting your client go out the door at the end of the session, quickly ask yourself if you have forgotten to do or ask something that will later come back and bite you. Make sure you have considered PODS. Could your client be **p**sychotic, **o**rganic (like a brain tumor that is primarily a physical cause of illness), **d**rug-affected/**d**epressed, or **s**uicidal? Is there some important information you have not gathered? Is that weapon still secure, as you were told earlier?

The last few minutes of the session can have special meaning. Sometimes, a client who wants to reveal something but does not want to deal with it will wait until they are holding onto the door to leave. Then they say, "By the way, I found out my husband has a second family. See you next week."

A client may see the end of the session as a signal that you believe you have helped them enough. It can feel like a mini termination. It is evidence that you don't recognize how much they are hurting. You are setting a limit on them and challenging their special neediness. You might see it as a vote of confidence that they can wait until their next visit to continue the work. Some clients, however, see it as you throwing them over for the next client. A client may be reminded of how their parents passed them over for a younger sibling.

Ideally, the end of the session might come with a synthesis of what your client has been saying, framed positively and reflecting your understanding. The end of the session is crowded with tasks, like reviewing directions, making an appointment, and maybe writing a prescription. Try to allow enough time for these tasks by paying attention to the clock. Make time to write your note. It bears repeating that if you don't write it down and document it, you have no evidence that it happened if you go to court.

Sometimes, clients will surprise you with what they can do.

Remember the waiting list effect, where the client starts feeling better just knowing they will see someone. Then there is the placebo effect, when someone feels better taking a sugar pill because they expect it to work. Don't demean these effects. The client needs every advantage possible.

You may have noticed that some clients who see novices do better than expected despite their severe illness because the novice did not know the client was not supposed to get that much better. Their collective hope inspired the client to make changes.

I had a revelation while studying neurological literature for my psychiatry board exams. I realized that I have attention deficit hyperactivity disorder. All those years, I thought it was as hard for everybody else as it was for me. I went to school during the Vietnam War era, and I had a low draft number. Failing out of medical school and getting killed in Vietnam was a palpable fear that kept me motivated. Oddly, I owe my career to the Vietnam War and to not knowing that finishing medical school was supposed to be almost unachievable for me.

Client progress may not be linear.

A client told me it might seem like she was going in circles with her growth. She said that, in fact, she was going around in spirals. She was still repeating behaviors but could now see them better from above.

In school, your grades reflected your progress. As a therapist, you might seek confirmation of your abilities by looking at your client's progress. They are not the same. Check yourself to be sure you are not unconsciously pressuring your client to get well. Sometimes, your clients may show no overt signs of improvement, but they may be gaining insight, as my client described it, in spirals. On other occasions, you are planting seeds that take time to bloom. Clients may also regress to regroup after an unusual stressor. Consider discussing your treatment and diagnosis with a supervisor or colleague when you feel your client is not progressing.

Remember, you may be a client's transitional object.

Your client benefits from you being a steady, consistent, dependable, separate person, just like a child can count on the teddy bear they use as a transitional object in their efforts to relate to a "non-me." When you feel that a client is kicking you around, remember that the teddy bear, though loved, is also dragged through the dirt. It is about persisting in being there for the client.

Some clients are adept at splitting care systems.

Some character-disordered clients can disrupt systems in a way that reflects their own dynamics.

Nursing staff used to come to me to explain that a particularly manipulative, impulsive patient would be too much for the staff to deal with and set limits on. Staff memories of her last hospitalization were widely different from each other, but all could agree that her stay had been disruptive to the therapeutic community.

I went to my director, explained what the nursing staff had told me, and asked if we could refuse the woman's admission. He put a limit on me and told me that he expected me to admit her, treat her, and help the staff. I returned to the staff and told them that I expected them to handle her and set limits on her. They returned to the patient and said they would admit her, but they expected her to control herself and abide by the limits. My boss realized the limits had to be set at all three levels.

Overdoing may be a defense.

Sometimes, clients with a parent who is a failure will resolve to not be like their parent. Because they have internalized part of that parent, they naturally worry about being just like them. They have a deep fear of falling apart and not functioning, like their parent who fell apart.

This fear makes objective success and accomplishment, as well as reassurance, very important. The client may be tired of having to be so aggressive and unconsciously wish to be passive. They may want to stop and relax. But they fear that passive wish because it feels like if they give in to it, they can never get back on the treadmill and will become their parent.

Sometimes, regression in the service of the ego is a necessary part of progress. In that situation, the client momentarily uses older coping techniques when under tremendous stress because it takes less effort. They need all their energy to regroup. Clients who must overdo it struggle to accept healthy regression.

People who overdo it also have trouble taking vacations. You may remember that going on vacation rates as a thirteen-point stress on the Social Readjustment Rating Scale, often called the Holmes and Rahe Stress Scale. Saul McLeod explains the Social Readjustment Rating Scale in Simply Psychology at this link: https://www.simplypsychology.org/srrs.html

Other times, overdoing it is a way of avoiding feelings. One client became depressed some months after losing her son. She had stayed busy and run away from the despair until she broke her leg and literally could not keep running.

In this chapter: I discussed the importance of not assuming things about your client or the nature of their progress. What you take for a given is not a given for them. They may fear the stigma of seeing you, the possibility of your disapproval if they tell you their secrets, or their belief that if they aren't busy, their minds will discover something disconcerting.

In the next chapter: I share my experience working with dissociating clients.

Chapter 32

Determine If Clients Have Dissociative Disease

My experience in working with people who have dissociative disease may not be representative. Nonetheless, I want to share things that appear true to my experience. You may be having sessions with an alter whose job is to see therapists. Look for history and behavioral clues that suggest early trauma. Alters have different roles and are triggered. Safety is paramount to clients with dissociative identity disorder.

Some of the most baffling clients I have treated have dissociative disease.

Not every child who is abused can dissociate. Being able to dissociate is a blessing at first, but the child may use that ability at other times until it becomes a reflex. I believe that alters (alternate identities) form over time to fulfill different tasks.

When the core personality (who was originally undivided and is as old as the body) can't tolerate being consciously there,

there is a switch. In an instant, an alter comes into consciousness instead. The client is said to have dissociated.

Sometimes, a therapist can witness a switch when there is a change in expression and mannerisms. If clients need to switch during a session, they sometimes run to the restroom.

The dissociative identity disorder diagnosis used to be called multiple personality disorder, but the name was changed to reflect the fact that the alternative identities are not fully formed, distinct personalities. Everyone does not dissociate to the same degree, and dissociative identity disorder is just one way in which dissociation manifests.

There may be alters who are of different ages. Their job is to hold the trauma memories of that age. A baby alter may represent the undefiled child, sort of like an artist might make a master of a record.

An aggressive alter may stand up for the core personality when bullied. A more sociable alter is in the body when intercourse occurs. Another alter might be more of a hermit.

Sometimes, the hermit hates being dragged around to social events, and the social alter hates the hermit for staying home. Sometimes, the less aggressive alters regret the violence the aggressive alter has done. These differences can lead to inner conflict, and there is an internal self-helper (termed an "ish") who may mediate in disputes. The therapist never sees the ish because the ish never manifests externally in the body consciousness, but other alters attest to its internal existence.

It seems like, untreated, the aggressive alter gets the upper hand, while the meek alters get bullied. As the core gives away more responsibility for coping with daily life, the core personality feels more depleted. Sometimes, the aggressive alter will complain that the core is such a wimp and never stands up for themselves.

Alters may talk to each other, and the client experiences hearing voices that don't speak to them but to each other. They may describe what sounds like what you hear when you first walk into a busy restaurant where lots of people are talking in the background.

Clients will lose time, and time will go by without them knowing what they did. They may move a cup and then ask someone else how it got there. They might remember nothing that was done or said. It depends on how far back they are from consciousness.

The most critical issue for a person with dissociative identity disorder is safety.

They cannot allow themselves to fully trust others for fear of their safety. Never think you are being trusted. Some alters watch you in the session. Every little behavior is scrutinized for threat and sincerity. You may not realize that you are treating someone with dissociative disease because the core personality has an alter whose job is to see therapists and doctors. The alter you are seeing is very responsible and rational, but they tell you about events that puzzle them. They have lost time and come into the body when an alter has caused a crisis. As you work with them, you are surprised that the same person can exhibit such different behaviors. They repeatedly feel like another alter has left them holding the bag for something they did not do.

Different events can trigger alters. Sometimes, manipulative partners will learn to trigger an alter to serve their purpose. On the other hand, in my limited experience, people with dissociative disease often marry people who are not threatening and can be outsmarted if necessary.

If you discover that your client has significant dissociative disease and you don't feel qualified to treat them, it may be challenging to find a therapist with the special training needed. Still, I urge you to keep looking because effective treatment can make such a difference in your client's life and the lives of their family members.

Effective treatment will involve teaching the client affective containment techniques and helping the core personality learn to blend instead of switching by accepting and working with alters while staying in the body. Sometimes, treatment involves disabling programming embedded by perpetrators.

Sometimes, using the mental construct of an inner safe place is useful in helping clients develop imagery that promotes inter-alter communication and a sense of safety.

In the *European Journal of Psychotraumatology*, Onno van der Hart's article explores this more. It is titled "The Use of Imagery in Phase 1 Treatment of Clients with complex dissociative disorders." https://pmc.ncbi.nlm.nih.gov/articles/ PMC3402145/

Helping clients cope with dissociation

Telling a client you suspect they have a dissociative identity disorder is ringing a bell that cannot be unrung. Some clients will be greatly relieved and tell you they have suspected something like this for a while. Others will be completely blindsided and overwhelmed. Some clients return the following week and display minor cuts on their arms where they have been punished for telling the therapist too much. Alters feel that their existence is threatened and can panic and act out.

It is essential to understand your dissociative client's life situation. Is there a support system that might help your client during the rough patches of therapy? Can your client financially sustain treatment long enough to make a difference? Would it make more sense to teach affective containment strategies and address more of the problems of daily life while slowly establishing a more stable setting for the long-term work? For example, some clients go back to school and gain job skills to afford long-term therapy. Others may move to a larger city with more treatment options.

On the other hand, are there circumstances that cause the alters to put your client in danger with risky behavior? Acting out, unprotected intercourse, and drug abuse put your client at risk and may force you to intervene immediately.

Clients can use the affective containment techniques you introduce early in therapy, along with the safe place, to help them cope with dissociation. It is a way to deal with triggers and can be tailored to each person's needs. When you introduce them to the safe place description through guided imagery, encourage clients to use their creativity to make it their own.

The ISSTD Adult Treatment Guidelines (2011 Revision) provide more details on the safe place and its features. I offer you the safe place description I was taught, which is based on these guidelines. It has evolved over the years, as some elements of the original description have been forgotten and others have been adapted.

When I use guided imagery, I tell clients that I am going to close my eyes and ask them to close theirs. I want to give them a sense of privacy by closing my eyes. I know that only the core personality can successfully incorporate the safe place, and the core is more likely to come into consciousness when they don't feel watched. Sometimes, the client takes my printed description with them to incorporate the safe place later on their own. It may take several tries. Here it is:

Imagine a circle of land surrounded by a wall of impenetrable light that goes up as far as you can see. Inside, you come upon an open field of several hundred yards. A sensor circles the inner perimeter. If a part crosses this sensor, it triggers three devices located on the top of the safe place.

These parts have an unobstructed view of everything that comes into the yard. One device announces to all in the safe place that a new part is entering. You can make the signal's sound any sound you like. Then there is a device that sends out strong magnetic pulses that can stop a malicious electronic device in its tracks. The third device is a water cannon that shoots water to immediately rust out any malicious mechanical device.

After you cross this inner perimeter, you see a large yard that has a playground for child parts. The front door of the safe place provides a view of the entire field and is made of plexiglass that cannot be broken.

There is no glass in the safe place, only unbreakable plexiglass. Because everything in the safe place runs on light, there is no need for electricity, so no one can be shocked.

There is a special entrance into the safe place for entering parts. A volunteer greets the entering part and helps them into a special pool. If the part is a baby, they are placed in a special basket that allows them to be washed safely. The pool is shallow so that no one can drown in it.

Being in the pool washes malicious programs off the part as they enter the switching place.

These programs may be things that a perpetrator told them or more sophisticated programming. This purification process protects parts in the safe place from contamination by malicious programming from an entering part. The switching place is kind of like a revolving door, and parts must go through it to enter after being washed.

Inside the safe place is an activity room with activities that a part might want to do, as well as a library of books and audio-visual items.

There is a large meeting room in the center of the safe place, and in this room is a large, round table with a place for every part. In each part's place are their favorite foods, which are replenished when eaten. The round table can be used for meals, meetings, and informal get-togethers. The table enlarges so there are always places available to newly entered parts. The round table symbolizes equality, respect, and acceptance. It also serves as a mechanism for cooperative problem-solving and discussion. In this room, there is a bank of computers that anyone can use at any time.

Each part has its own room, which can be decorated and furnished the way they like. People of different ages may decorate their rooms in ways that reflect their age, such as a teenager, a college student, or a young child. They have personal computers in their rooms they can use to send messages to each other and to the core. No one can enter a part's room except the part. Parts hang out in the hallways and common rooms. A part's room is treated as their sacred space.

The core personality's room is slightly bigger than a part's room because it houses the master computer. The core uses this computer to communicate with the parts. The core periodically checks their computer's bulletin board to read parts' opinions and requests, keep track of what is going on, and respond.

As well as providing a framework for functioning, the safe place has a nourishing atmosphere of cooperation, acceptance, and emotional warmth.

Working with "multiples" has parallels with working with "uni-brains." For example, just as you would encourage a uni-brain to accept themselves, you encourage multiples' parts to accept each other. You may be using a different language or internal mental constructs, but the goal of self-acceptance is the same.

You may help parts work together to reach a compromise solution as they solve problems. With uni-brains, you use a parallel construct to help the ego modulate the id and superego to better regulate drive activity. As you work with parts and they begin to cooperate with each other, there can be excitement over what they are learning and what they can do when they work together.

Before treatment, when something stressful was going on, the core would have a split second when they felt uncomfortable and were about to switch and throw an alter into the situation while they escaped consciousness. Teaching the core to recognize that split-second feeling and resist the urge to switch is an essential part of therapy.

As the core personality learns to accept the parts and the parts learn to work together, it becomes easier for the core to welcome parts into co-consciousness in a blend. Part of the goal of therapy is to develop the core's ability to stay in the body as a conscious participant in what is going on and to invite parts to blend with the core, standing united in the face of adversity. Rather than switching, the core affects a blend, can utilize the parts' skills, and remains aware of what is happening without dissociating. *United We Stand: A Book for People with Multiple Personalities* by Eliana Gil illustrates this and is written as a children's book for child parts so they can better understand.

In this chapter: I gave you an overview of dissociative disease.

In the next chapter: I offer a glimpse into the world of clients with autism.

Chapter 33

Decide If Clients Are Autistic

Autistic people differ significantly from each other, which contributes to their baffling qualities and means that the material in this chapter may not apply to your clients.

I encourage you to view my YouTube video called *Misconceptions About People with High-Functioning Autism.* https://www.youtube.com/watch?v=hLn6D4NujVU

In the time since this video was recorded, the term *high-functioning autism* has been dropped. Autistic people are now referred to as having autistic spectrum disorder and the number 1, 2, or 3. The number describes how much support they might need and their capacity for independent function. The same autistic person may have a different number at different times. Added effort and outside support may enable them to function differently at other times. The number 1 designation is for clients who typically require the least support and can mask their autistic thinking for extended periods, resulting in the appearance of more independence.

In a July 2025 MDEdge article, Patricia Wendling discussed research published that same month in *Nature Genetics*. She noted that researchers had identified four clinically distinct autism subtypes and their underlying genetic signals. This research may lead to further changes in how autistic people are described. https://www.mdedge.com/psychiatry?summaryguid=2025a1000isl&ecd=WNL_PSYCH_250728_mdedge&uac=3006SK&sso=true

Here are some pieces of the autism puzzle that my clients and the literature have shown me. As you read about these pieces, ask yourself whether they fit with what you know and your experiences.

Consider these two generalizations about people with autism.

It is hard to generalize about people with autism, but I agree with two generalizations that appear somewhat broadly held. First, I believe it is true when they say, "When you have met one person with autism, you have met just one person with autism, and you cannot generalize from that one experience."

Second, I agree that ordinary people do many of the same things that autistic people do, but autistic people do those things most of the time. For example, ordinary people often have drinks with them. Many clients with autism, if they like drinks, keep something to drink with them almost all the time. They feel uncomfortable without them.

On the other hand, some autistic clients will forget to eat or drink for long periods if they are absorbed by something they are doing and are not prompted by others.

Neural wiring and neurotransmitter function appear to be different in clients with autism.

Much remains to be known about autism, but I am going to side with those who say autistic clients have variations in neural wiring and neurotransmitter function. I think of autistic brains as being different rather than being ordinary brains with deficits. I see it as analogous to how some computers are Apple systems and others are disc operating systems. One would say they are different, but not that one is sick and the other is well. Each has its strengths and weaknesses.

My clients tell me they can't imagine something new without connecting it to what they already know. Having to recite poems for my senior English teacher, I would get halfway through and forget the following line. Then I'd have to go back and start over to get my brain to remember the following line. A friend singing the Lord's Prayer in church forgot the words and had to go back from the beginning and sing it all over again. Similarly, if you interrupt an autistic client's train of thought, they have to start over. They may get irritated at you for interrupting them.

Long before starting a behavior, some clients may have to sit on their bed, lost in thought.

Because their sense of taste, smell, or hearing may differ, they respond differently to different sensations. Autistic clients may detect when food has spoiled before others do. They may love the sound of an egg cracking, the crunch of their shoes on snow, or the taste of just one kind of Coke in just one type of bottle, drunk down to a certain point at a specific temperature. They can sense meaningful differences.

Imagine that you have a keen sense of smell. One sunny spring morning, you walk outside to the sudden scent of gardenias. It is a brief but intense experience. Now imagine an experience that is just that intense and all-consuming, but it is a dead skunk in your front yard. You would wish you could not smell so well, but your keen sense of smell is with you in both instances. Autistic clients have described their experience of daily reality as being inescapably intense like that.

For some clients, things must necessarily connect directly from past knowledge and have what appears to them to be a logical connection. They can't brush their teeth before showering. They can't floss before brushing. If they are going to a job interview, they have a million little things to do in a set sequence, and if they can't do each one, they may just shut down. They shut down in a way that neurotypical people cannot do. It is a different neurological experience. It can feel like they simply don't exist or that the activity requiring their effort has lost its meaning.

Other autistic clients may not develop routines despite their best efforts. They describe it as though their circadian rhythm is off, and their eating, sleep, and work habits are never consistent or predictable. They set multiple alarms to rouse them from what they describe as profound sleep.

I have seen clients who don't exactly see themselves as having a body. It is not clear whether this is a manifestation of autism or part of a comorbid dissociative disease. Pain and sickness may surprise and irritate them. They have to deal with a body when they see themselves more as a kind of disembodied consciousness. They may feel annoyed at having to choose clothes for this body or alarmed when others are attracted to it and they must deal with that person. Parents may be distressed that their child is not interested in seeing a doctor for this body. The client may be indifferent to this body, as it doesn't truly represent who they feel they are.

Some people have described this kind of disembodied consciousness as being like a camera whose function is to watch and record but was not really made for participating, even though it can. But if it is engaging, it can't perform its natural function.

When I heard this camera analogy, I thought of the family therapist who allows himself to participate in the family process but then pulls back to observe what he has just been involved in. The family therapist is not there to belong to the family. He is an outside observer who helps but is keenly aware of his separateness. Yet the family therapist can belong to his own family, while the autistic person may feel belonging is not natural for them. The autistic person's lack of connection makes observation all the more necessary.

One client further clarified this. They noted that while observation is an essential part of the ability to understand and adapt or mimic the world around them, the autistic person's brain does not allow them to completely focus on what others might see as relevant.

When they find themselves in a crucial situation requiring correct observation, it requires much effort. Observation becomes natural only when their interest is sparked. Unfortunately, they find themselves interested in things that are usually not pertinent, and their interests feel more like distractions. On other occasions, their creative, involuntary, outside-the-box thinking has rewarded humanity with remarkable discoveries.

In her Netflix special called *Nannette* and her TED Talk, Hannah Gadsby shared her insights into what it is like to be autistic and what her thought process is like. You can find her TED Talk at https://www.ted.com/speakers/hannah_gadsby

Being with other people can be stressful for autistic clients.

An occasional client will have an extreme fear of being seen. An example of being seen might be if a girl bought a new dress she really liked, and another girl made a dismissive remark about it. It is not simply being noticed but being noticed and receiving a cutting remark.

When your client talks to you, their eyes may go all over the room to avoid observing that you are looking at them critically. If they do feel the need to show they are listening by staring at your eyes, it quickly tires them. Being noticed in a social situation is stressful because it may require them to decide what a normal person would do and then try to do that.

One client told me she awakens each day looking at the ceiling. If the ceiling is familiar, she knows where she is. Then she thinks, *Who am I?* then, *What am I doing here?* Then, she follows a series of steps that may take half an hour before she gets out of bed. She says she feels like Bill Murray in *Groundhog Day* or Drew Barrymore in *50 First Dates.*

Autistic clients have told me they grew up wishing they could be normal but eventually realized they could not. They could mimic normal behaviors with great effort and only for brief periods. They hoped the people they loved would accept that they were okay as autistic people and love them as they were, without wanting them to be normal or making being normal a condition for being loved. Some have told me they struggle with accepting what they feel is the harsh reality that their loved ones can never do that entirely.

A client explained that she looked forward to being alone, not because she particularly enjoyed being alone, but because she liked not being overwhelmed. Whenever she interacted with the neurotypical world, she required downtime to recover. When she closed the door to her room, she could restrict stimulation and did not have to continually respond to situations or people. She felt free to stim without someone judging her. (Stimming involves doing repetitive, purposeless, self-stimulating behaviors, such as hand flapping, rocking, or repeating sounds, to cope with stress. Not everyone who stims is autistic, and not all autistic people stim.) She said that the entire time she was out, she looked forward to the next time she could close the door behind her.

Hearing that, I thought of the family therapy concept of the embassy room. The family is asked to designate a room where members can seek refuge, similar to an asylum-seeking immigrant. There are no electronics, and no one talks in the embassy room. They are silent and sit until they want to come out. Having an embassy room might reduce autistic clients' need to elope and vanish from the area to regroup.

Sometimes, by the time your autistic client meets you, they have developed PTSD from the trauma of repeatedly failing to meet the demands of living in the neurotypical world. The very act of trying recreates the triggering situation, and they get burned out. This burnout raises the risk of suicide.

When autistic clients are with someone who is in severe physical pain, they may immediately feel that pain in their body. It is a visceral reaction, unlike the thinking process of neurotypicals, which results in empathetic thoughts. Ordinary situations might not provoke this chameleon-like response to the environment, but autistic people are aware of this vulnerability to the feelings of others.

Their behaviors make sense when you realize that their experience of reality differs from yours.

Clients with OCD and autism may want to do things a certain way.

The client with OCD is rigid and becomes bothered and anxious when things are not done a certain way.

Autistic clients may not have any anxiety about doing something different. It is just not logical for them, and they don't want to do it because it makes little sense. When an autistic person must pick food from a menu, they often choose the same one each time. It is logical for them to select the same one because they know it. They may crave what they already know to be good because they know eating it will again be comforting. They think it is illogical to pick one they don't know because they don't know if they like it.

Autistic clients look like they are in a rut because they may eat the same things each day and not explore other choices. Their life may seem dull, but for the autistic person, life is filled with a persistent examination of minutiae. The tiniest details of how things fit together intrigue autistic people, and they will research a topic at length on the internet.

This different way of thinking seems like a computer whose memory is almost filled up and must go through everything bit by bit along the same path to find the needed item. So, while the autistic brain might process quickly, it has more to process to respond.

You may sometimes run into conflict over something an autistic client doesn't want to change. Family members may tell you about similar disputes. It might involve the client giving up a habit that is detrimental to their well-being. Or they may need to conform to expected behavior that could result in what society defines as a successful life.

When talking about having been asked to give up drinking Coke because of its effect on her teeth, one client eloquently described how what seems trivial to others could be life-sustaining for her. She said that the comforts that remained for her were small because they were all she could cling to. She said she clung tighter to them over time because the number of those things dwindled, taking the joy of life with them. The little things became increasingly more important to hold onto. These were far from trivial to her because she realized what a difference a little joy could make, and she realized how profoundly necessary that little bit of joy was to her existence. I realized that asking her to give up Coke was tantamount to taking away a child's only doll. That tempered my natural tendency to advocate for all things healthy.

Explore the pathological (or extreme) demand avoidance (PDA) concept and see if it applies to your clients. PDA is an unusual resistance to ordinary social demands and even to demands the client wants for themselves. The Extreme Demand Avoidance Questionnaire, which was used with children, has been adapted for use with adults. You can find it here https://embrace-autism.com/eda-qa/

When you read about PDA, you will be told that going along with others' demands feels like a threat to the autistic person's autonomy. I would go a step further and say that giving in can make them feel like they are in outer space and are allowing a hole to be pierced in the spacesuit whose integrity protects their very existence.

Because some of the same parts of the brain affected by autism are also affected by ADHD, they share some common symptoms. Some autistic people have additional symptoms that meet the criteria for both autism and ADHD. Most people with ADHD have no autistic symptoms.

Sometimes, clients with autism who have been mistreated as children did not recognize the abuse as abuse because they did not know it could be different until they saw families who were not abusive.

Autistic clients use various behaviors to communicate their feelings.

People with autism want others to listen closely to what they say and their explanations of why they want to do something a certain way. They may infodump as a way of showing affection by describing in great detail an area of their intense interest with no clue that they have exceeded your ability to listen.

You will learn about penguin pebbling and other ways people with autism express their wish to connect with others when you read an excellent discussion by Myth@neurowonderful at this Stimpunks Foundation site: https://stimpunks.org/2022/01/22/the-five-neurodivergent-love-languages-2/

Your autistic client may benefit from knowing about the Stimpunks Foundation. According to the foundation, Stimpunks is "a 501 (c)(3) nonprofit built by and for neurodivergent and disabled people." It was "forged in the quest for survival and inclusion."

People with autism have much to offer and can enrich our lives with their unique skills and different take on the world.

Compromise is key in working with autistic clients.

Therapists, family members, friends, and partners may find that interacting productively with a person with autism can be awkward. Even though there is great variation from client to client, I would like to suggest some broad concepts that might help.

First, accept that your client has an autistic brain and what the implications are. You could demonstrate your acceptance by dimming your office lights to accommodate their light sensitivity. If they have problems with noise, reduce office noise. If they have problems with crowds, schedule them for times when the office is less crowded. If they have problems leaving the house, see them remotely first.

Look for comorbid depression and attention deficit hyperactivity disorder. Successfully treating them could help lay a foundation for a more positive therapeutic relationship. You want to demonstrate that you are useful and that something can be changed. Look for the low-lying fruit to pick first and, in that way, help dispel feelings of being stuck.

If they have trouble with processing, it will be important to speak slowly and check with them to make sure they understand what you have said. You may need longer appointment times so you have time to explain things in more detail.

Because of their tendency toward pathological demand avoidance, it is more important than ever to repeatedly align what you are doing in therapy with what your client has told you they want to accomplish. They need to know that it is their therapy and not one imposed by neurotypical authorities. This is particularly frustrating when you or a family member feels a more urgent health-related matter should come first.

Always keeping autonomy in mind, please collaborate on developing small steps toward a realistic goal that your client agrees is logical. Some autistic clients have a way of ignoring necessary responsibilities, so you may need to survey the entire picture to make sure nothing more urgent is overlooked.

Ironically, your ability to compromise is even more crucial when you're working with clients who have difficulty compromising. You have less ability to influence client behavior, and you, like their parent, must remember that you are doing your best.

Part of doing your best is listening carefully to autistic people because what they are telling you about how they experience reality is different from what you expect. You have to continually question your assumptions.

Identify what brings joy to your autistic client and foster it. Celebrate each small victory. While trying to have serenity about what you can't control, don't overlook the progress you have helped the client make. Just as their parents should take note of what they have been able to do, so should you.

There is controversy in the field of autism treatment over whether treatment should be geared to helping clients mask and fit in or helping them accept their differences and live a life that, though it is more restricted than society finds successful, is also more survivable. In the face of the need for their own financial support, it may be hard to determine what is reasonable to expect from any one autistic person.

In this chapter: I explained that differences in neural wiring and neurotransmitters result in widely varying expressions of neuroatypicality. These variations may be in differences in sensory abilities, expression of affection, and skills. The client with autism has a different experience of reality. The atypical clients who can mask their symptoms and mimic neurotypicals find masking can exhaust them and lead to despair. When they experience PDA, it can frustrate their family as well.

In the next chapter: I talk about issues around medication. You may prescribe medication, or you may work with a prescriber. But either way, you are in a medical minefield if your client is taking medication. I'll look at some mines in that field, including noncompliant clients, less-than-ideal work settings, paperwork, neglected contraception, and drug side effects. Clients may be slow metabolizers, experience drug withdrawal, or experience intolerable motor restlessness that exacerbates their anxiety. The next chapter will highlight how establishing routine procedures, documenting treatment, being available, and getting help when needed can help you navigate that minefield.

Part 5

BE CAREFUL TRAVERSING
THE MEDICAL MINEFIELD

Even if you are not a prescriber, you may still be in a medical minefield if your client has medical issues, takes medication, or needs to take medication but has misconceptions about it, or if you must collaborate with a prescriber. This section addresses some of these, and the final chapter of this section points out some surprising associations.

Chapter 34

Anticipate Difficulties When Clients Are Taking Medication

Establishing best practices includes discussing contraception with childbearing clients. Don't walk into the minefield without the protective armor of excellent documentation, consistent availability, and the help of colleagues when needed.

Get help providing treatment when you need it.

Hubris is dangerous. Don't let pride or discomfort stop you from asking for help from unlikely sources. Occasionally, you will feel you are between a rock and a hard place in dealing with what to prescribe or do. You may be choosing between the lesser of several evils, but there is no logical choice. In those instances, admit that you just don't know. You must call around until you get enough information to take a calculated risk. That means doing more literature research or talking to peers. You could speak to the pharmaceutical company expert on call for the drugs involved. (Their phone number is in the physician's desk reference by drug manufacturer.) Consider calling drug representatives, past teachers, or former classmates. Or ask for a formal consultation.

I was lucky to have an ongoing relationship with a coworker who was a doctor of pharmacy and a researcher. I have called other pharmacists who have been happy to help. Pharmacists have a customer base drawn from multiple providers prescribing the same medication. Pharmacists get a larger volume of feedback about medication side effects. Clients also may be less reluctant to complain to their pharmacist than to their provider. This makes pharmacists a valuable source of information, even though that information might be anecdotal.

It is okay to feel embarrassed and uncomfortable, ask for undeserved favors, and inconvenience busy people who don't have the time to talk to you to get the information you need to decide. Remember that you don't know the nature of what you don't know, which can come back and bite you and the client. Sometimes, being insistent is called for.

Be available.

Take it seriously when clients complain that they cannot contact you quickly. Look at the entire communication chain. My first secretary made it difficult for clients to reach me and seemed to enjoy having the power to say no. She saw it as protecting me and as part of her job. Clients who believe in you are more likely to believe in your prescribed medication. If they think you don't care because you are hard to get, they are unlikely to take your medication.

Be ready to adapt to situations that are less than ideal.

I was on call for my unit as a first-year resident. One patient was constipated. I looked up all the laxatives in the physician's desk reference and selected what I thought was the best one. The unit said they did not have that laxative. Doing more research, I came up with the second-best laxative. They didn't have that one either. Finally, I asked what they had in their medicine cabinet, and they told me about the laxative they had.

That was a lesson in the practical. I went from the theoretical to the real. My adaptation experience was particularly helpful when I worked in community mental health centers with clients who had limited resources. I had to use available samples there, but they were not my first choices.

You may encounter manufacturing or supply chain problems with a particular medication. When I worked at Georgia College and State University, the local pharmacies ran out of long-acting Adderall. So prescribers in the area substituted another medication whose supply eventually ran out. At some point, before I prescribed any psychostimulant, I had to call pharmacies and ask them to give me an idea of what they had in stock. I was back to asking what was in the medicine cabinet and making adjustments.

Establishing and following procedures may reduce the risk of medical-legal problems.

Develop your usual informed consent process to ensure that you are less likely to leave anything out. Document that you have given your usual informed consent. In addition, you want to document that you asked if the client had questions and answered them to their satisfaction. Recording this shows a collaboration because you are not just handing the client a printed form about the medication. Do this because clients forget you have informed them. When they testify in court that you never told them that, you will have no defense if you don't document it.

I am told that juries may forgive you for making a mistake but will always rule against you if they have any sign that you tampered with the record. Make your notes when you see the client. Remember, the metadata on the computer can be made available in court to show when you wrote the document.

Your notes should convey the courses of action you considered, why you did not choose the ones you rejected, and the reasoning behind your choice.

Accept that paperwork is an essential part of excellent treatment.

Requesting past medical records is good practice and the standard of care. It can help you anticipate difficulties with medication. When you see someone else's patient in consultation, write a report to the referring provider, thanking them for the referral and explaining your findings and recommendations. You want to express your willingness to discuss matters further and provide your contact information so they can easily reach you.

When referring a client for consultation or further treatment, send your records and a referral letter after you have the client's informed consent. Your records should explain your thinking and recommendations. Make sure your client has enough medication to last until they can be seen. Let your client know you are available in the interim and how they can reach you. Document that you have told them about your availability.

You may end up writing for additional medication if there is a hold-up. In this way, the client does not feel abandoned and there is continuity of care.

Additional phone calls, calls to pharmacies, contact with referring providers, and calls to families or other people treating your client can be time-consuming and are not usually budgeted for in your schedule. They are no less part of the treatment. This extra effort shows the client that you care about them and their treatment.

The need for effective contraception cannot be overemphasized to medicated clients.

It is essential that you educate your female clients about their need for effective contraception while taking medication. One day each year, our country celebrates the men who believe that a condom by itself is a 100 percent effective form of contraception. That day is called Father's Day.

Document your discussion about contraception, and keep reminding clients about it. They need to know about the risk of fetal harm associated with their particular medication. Also know which medications lower oral contraceptives' effectiveness.

I wrote *Exploring Your Unplanned Pregnancy: Single Motherhood, Adoption, and Abortion Questions and Resources* to provide women with an opportunity to ask important questions and offer education and resources. Since 2015, some resources have changed, but the questions that help them through the decision-making process are still valid. Visit jeffduffeymdbooks.com to learn more about this book.

Drug studies have limitations.

If you have a client taking medication or if you prescribe medication, it is worth noting a few observations about drug studies. Drug companies would not want to risk giving a drug to a pregnant woman who might incur fetal damage. So they are less likely to include women in drug studies. Instead, they use lab animals to determine fetal risk. Women sometimes respond differently to medication than men taking the same medication.

Drug studies often exclude clients with comorbid illnesses from studies because their comorbid illness is a variable that might cause a different outcome. It would not be clear whether the outcome was related to the comorbid illness or the medication. As a result, information about how the drug interacts with clients with a comorbid illness may be lacking.

When a pharmaceutical company has determined that a drug would be helpful, they do dose-ranging studies to determine how much medication is required for it to be safe and effective.

Let's say a study was done, and the maximum dose given of drug X was 100 mg. When the FDA approved the drug, it did not have any proof of what drug X does above 100 mg daily. So it does not approve the use of drug X above 100 mg a day. Using drug X above 100 mg a day is an off-label use. A prescriber may believe it takes more than 100 mg a day of drug X for a fast-metabolizer of drug X to get an effective blood level. Off-label prescribing requires careful consideration of the risks and benefits. It may require a literature search to find what other providers who have tried the drug at higher doses have discovered.

A prescriber might also prescribe an off-label medication for an indication that the FDA has not approved. The FDA cannot approve an indication if it has not been adequately studied and proven effective. The absence of FDA approval may mean that the FDA has reviewed studies and found that the medication was ineffective or had unacceptable side effects. Sometimes, it just means that the FDA has not yet studied the product.

When drug Y came to the US, it was said to be one of the most popular drugs used to treat depression in Europe. The FDA does not accept research done in other countries. The company that made drug Y looked at the antidepressant market in the US and decided to spend money on research to get drug Y approved to treat OCD. It was approved only for OCD since no studies were done regarding antidepressant effectiveness. Thus, a prescriber using drug Y to treat depression would use it off-label, despite it being used extensively in Europe to treat depression.

Different prescribers have different philosophies about prescribing new medications. Some wait until the medication has been around for a while because they know that some severe side effects occur rarely. Also, drug studies may not have had enough subjects for the side effects to come up.

Your client's experience of side effects may not be generalized to others.

Anticipate patient variation to avoid difficulties with clients taking medication. There is a human tendency to avoid prescribing a medication that has caused a significant side effect in a client, even though the prescriber has read the medication literature and knows the drug has a low incidence of that side effect in the general population.

I had a thin female client who had a seizure on an antidepressant. She had not been drinking much liquid and had become somewhat dehydrated. That raised the level of the medication in her blood. She drank alcohol, which lowered the seizure threshold. She was thin, so she had little total body water to dilute the medication to begin with. The dose of medication I prescribed was a starter dose that the literature suggested has a seizure incidence of about one in a thousand. The combination of factors resulted in her having a seizure, even at the low dose. She may also have been a slow metabolizer of the medication. I did not have genetic testing to know.

After that experience, I thought twice about prescribing that medication, even though I know the seizure risk is ordinarily low.

Slow metabolizers may have side effects at a standard medication dose.

If you have a client who, on the surface, appears very finicky about medication, seems to lack the willingness to tolerate side effects, and seems to have side effects at what you think are minuscule doses, don't assume they are just being difficult or a help-rejecting complainer. They might be a slow metabolizer. As discussed earlier, genetic testing might confirm this and give you a better idea of what works.

You might need to lower the dose in a slow metabolizer and raise the dose in a fast metabolizer. If they have a problem with the SERT transporter, you may have to use a different type of medication to avoid them becoming suicidal. As mentioned earlier, genetic testing can alert you to this. Please pay attention to what your client says about their response and don't think concretely about dose recommendations.

A side effect may be riskier in specific groups.

A medication that might be safe for one person to take may be dangerous for another. For example, medicines that can cause postural hypotension can be risky for older clients who are at risk of falls or may have less vascular tone.

Clients who metabolize medication slowly will have a higher blood level than expected. Even a low dose of sedating medication could impair driving. A discussion about driving should be part of your usual informed consent process. Sometimes, prohibiting a client's driving is clinically indicated. If you fail to restrict a client from driving and they have an accident while taking the medication you prescribed, you are at risk of malpractice.

Consider each of your client's symptoms before you dismiss any.

Some clients exaggerate symptoms and essentially cry wolf. Even those who frequently cry wolf can have a significant, legitimate illness. There may be some legitimate symptoms in the collage of symptoms they complain about. Disease complexes also exist but may not be fully defined yet. (For example, I suspect we will see non-celiac gluten hypersensitivity gaining respect as a factor in multi-system illness.)

Men and other women tend to discount women's opinions in our culture. I have found that women are more aware of their bodies and more observant than men. When your female client expresses concern about something she observed, please take what she says seriously. She may help you catch something you overlooked or see it more accurately. Dismissing women's observations results in needless suffering and lost lives.

Having one diagnosis does not protect you from having another. You might expect a lack of motivation in a person with schizophrenia to be another one of their negative symptoms. Instead, it could be caused by anemia.

Motor restlessness/agitation and suicidal thinking are a dangerous combination.

When you have a client who is having suicidal thoughts, giving medication that increases motor restlessness or agitation can be dangerous. You may be more familiar with antipsychotics causing motor restlessness, but some more activating antidepressants can cause restlessness and agitation as well.

Let your client know that medication phase effects may eventually pass.

Some medications have phase effects. A phase effect is part of the main effect of the drug. For example, there can be a several-day dysphoric phase when clients first take Zoloft (sertraline) because of a transient drop in dopamine. If the client does not know about transient phase effects, they will be put off when they go through this dysphoric period, if it happens. You can anticipate difficulties with these phase adverse effects by including this information in your early client education.

If you have a scored pill, one-half of the active medication will be in each half. If you halve an unscored pill, all the active ingredients could be in one half and not the other. If you cannot get around halving an unscored pill, have the client take the other half of the same pill the next day. This way, they will have received the full dose within the forty-eight-hour period. Don't let the client halve multiple pills at the same time.

When a dentist injects Novocain, they administer a small amount and allow the tissue to adjust and become numb. Then they inject more. They don't inject it as fast as they can.

A medication is more likely to have side effects if the dose is raised too rapidly and the body does not have a chance to adjust. On the other hand, if the medication is introduced too slowly, the client may not see the beneficial effects soon enough and will want to stop the medication.

Don't forget the carrier protein.

Some medications compete with vitamins for the same carrier protein. So you may have to supplement vitamins when certain medications are taken at specific doses.

Ask yourself if the symptoms are a recurrence or medication withdrawal.

When a client stops medication suddenly, you may not be able to determine whether symptoms are related to a rebound or the reemergence of the underlying, incompletely treated illness. Know how long the client has been on the medication and how closely the symptoms resemble the associated discontinuation syndrome.

Look for unexpected drug withdrawal.

Sometimes, people you would not think have a drinking or drug problem actually do have one. When these people are in an accident or have surgery, they may have told no one about their usual alcohol or drug intake. When their withdrawal symptoms emerge, the symptoms may at first seem to be part of another illness. Have a high index of suspicion when someone suddenly loses control of their intake. You could be seeing drug or alcohol withdrawal.

Patient education and adherence are crucial for clients taking anticonvulsants.

If you have a client who is taking an anticonvulsant, the anticonvulsant raises the seizure threshold, so it is harder to have a seizure. If they suddenly stop the anticonvulsant, there is a rebound lowering of the seizure threshold that puts them at risk for a seizure. Your client may forget what you told them about not running out of their anticonvulsant or suddenly stopping it.

It may feel like you are infantilizing the client if you oversee too closely that they're taking the medication, but you cannot risk them having a seizure. They could be driving, swimming, bathing, climbing a ladder, or engaging in other risky activities.

So, as you prescribe medication, ensure that they have enough, especially if you are going out of town. Clients are sometimes reluctant to call the on-call doctor. If you have a young or irresponsible client or one with a poor compliance history, enlist a family member to watch.

Clients taking Lamictal (lamotrigine) require special considerations.

If a client misses several days of Lamictal and doesn't start over with the small starting dose, they are putting themselves at risk for Stevens-Johnson syndrome, which can be life-threatening. The Mayo Clinic discusses it here: https://www.mayoclinic.org/diseases-conditions/stevens-johnson-syndrome/symptoms-causes/syc-20355936

It may be inconvenient to call pharmacies on the weekend or go the extra mile, but the consequences of not doing so are too significant. You may be tempted to set limits, but this is not the time.

It is always important to document the informed consent you give a client. But with Lamictal, it is critical that you document what you told them about rash risk and how to minimize it by taking the medication correctly and alerting you immediately if they have a rash. Informed consent is not a single event but an ongoing process of educating and reminding the client and documenting what you have said. Some medications need less monitoring. Lamictal is not one of them.

In this chapter: I reminded you that things are not always how they seem. Clients metabolize medications differently than expected. They neglect to take birth control. Drug-induced motor restlessness can aggravate feelings of frantic hopelessness. Drug studies don't tell the entire story. Clients go into unexpected drug withdrawal. These are all good reasons to have established best practices in delivering care.

In the next chapter: I home in on misconceptions clients have about medication.

Chapter 35

Correct Clients' Misconceptions About Taking Medication

Prejudice and lack of education about medication may lead to nonadherence.

Taking antidepressants is not like taking aspirin.

When a client takes aspirin for a headache and the headache goes away, they stop the medication. It makes sense to clients to stop an antidepressant when they are no longer depressed. It is best if you repeatedly educate them about the need to continue taking the medication until their brain has healed. Different clinicians have different ideas about how long that is, but most would say it is long after the end of symptoms.

Stopping medication taken for depression may be dangerous.

Sometimes, you can't risk rebound depression when people stop antidepressants or experience discontinuation syndrome. Sometimes, people aren't motivated enough or they're too depressed to pick up the next prescription. They may be accustomed to having others do tasks for them and are not responsible enough. Perhaps they have forgotten your instructions or are ambivalent about taking the medication because it nauseated them. When you see the patient, ask yourself how dangerous their reaction would be if they missed medication. Would they be suicidal? Do you need to go the extra mile to ensure that they continue their medication?

Medicine is dosed to reach a therapeutic blood level, but clients think it reflects the severity of their illness.

Another misconception about medication that you need to correct is the belief that taking a higher dose means the client is sicker. They need to understand that dosage is about getting a therapeutic blood level and not how ill they are. Some clients feel God loves them more if they take the smallest dose possible. They feel that if they just had more faith, they would not need medication. They don't believe that God may work through medication.

Clients may use others to speak for them.

Sometimes, when a client tells you someone else does not want them taking medication, they are putting it on that other person. The client might not want to take the medication.

Your client's priorities may not be your own.

A client told me she had never felt better since starting Prozac, and she wanted me to reduce the dose. She said her husband was an alcoholic, and she had to be on guard. But the Prozac made her too relaxed and happy. Safety was more important to her than her happiness.

Some clients feel that taking medication is a mark against them.

Some people feel that medication is a crutch. Others believe that if they improve on medication, they don't get full credit for getting better. Clients who feel that taking medication is a blemish may insist on a medication they take only once daily. These are the same kind of people who insist that their child get a patch rather than need the school nurse to give them their psychostimulant in the middle of the day.

Other clients view medication as food they have bought and can't let go to waste.

One seventy-eight-year-old client complained bitterly about an aggravating side effect. She was relieved when I agreed to stop the medication and gave her a prescription for a different drug. I asked her to come back in two weeks to see how the new medication was working and adjust the dose. When she returned, she had not switched her medication. She explained she did not want to waste the remaining pills, so she'd continued the first medication. The Great Depression had touched her family. She had learned that if she threw something out, she might regret it when she needed it later.

Clients may be misleading.

When prescribing medication, it's essential to know if your client is following the instructions accurately. Clients may lie to you for many reasons, so it would be helpful to read *Never Be Lied to Again* by David J. Lieberman. I was so impressed by this book that I gave a copy to each of my daughters for Christmas because they were dating.

Sometimes, companies exaggerate the therapeutic effectiveness of their product. Understanding statistics and how to read journal articles may help you avoid being misled.

Encourage clients to pursue adequate treatment for their relatives.

You can support your clients by helping them identify their family members' physical illnesses and helping them obtain treatment. However, remember that you have a partial picture. It is no substitute for an adequate evaluation by another provider. Encourage your client to get help for their relatives. Also, you don't want to give out advice to friends and neighbors because you may inadvertently create a doctor-patient relationship that could put you at medical-legal risk.

In this chapter: I provided a short listing of client misconceptions about medication. You would like to see clients take medicine as prescribed, consult you before reducing or changing it, allow you to raise it to a therapeutic blood level, and taper it when no longer needed. Client education that anticipates the difficulties in doing this may prevent later problems.

In the next chapter: I cover topics that have only one thing in common: They may come as surprises.

Chapter 36

Recognize These Associations in Medicine

This chapter contains miscellaneous clues that might explain various medical situations.

When you have a client with odd symptoms, consider these explanations.

There are symptom combinations and diagnoses that you don't see very often, but having them in the back of your mind might help you solve a puzzle. When you see odd symptoms, ask yourself if it is depersonalization, dissociative disease, unacknowledged cannabis use, or odd medication side effects. Consider whether it might be a micro psychotic episode, autism, latent schizophrenia, or methamphetamine use. Think about secondary gain, a conversion symptom, or symptoms that are better explained by cultural beliefs.

Some antibiotics are associated with transient depression.

I have had clients who were doing well suddenly complain that they were having driving suicidal thoughts that they find disturbing. They were taking certain antibiotics that have been known to induce suicidal thinking. If a client tells you they are feeling suicidal for no reason, you should ask them if they have recently started a new medication.

Don't forget odd sources of intoxication.

Another odd connection happens when psychotic clients drink excessive amounts of coffee to counteract the sedating effect of major tranquilizers. They then show heightened anxiety and other signs of caffeine intoxication. Clients can also develop water intoxication from drinking too much water. Look for signs of hyponatremia.

Dyes and fillers may be the source of an allergy.

I had a client who broke out with allergic rashes to multiple antidepressant medications. I was puzzled because these drugs had different mechanisms of action. Finally, I realized that each medication had the same specific color dye on the coating. I found a medication that did not have that dye, and the patient responded without having an allergic reaction.

Lab work can be a double-edged sword.

If you order lab work, ensure that it gets back to you and does not sit in your mailbox or get placed in a stack somewhere you don't see. Failure to review and act on lab work can be grounds for malpractice if what was missed leads to an adverse outcome.

How your client responds to coffee may tell you something.

You may suspect that your client is a slow metabolizer on the 1A2 path if they become very jittery with coffee or experience insomnia after drinking it. Coffee is metabolized on that path.

Heat exhaustion is a real risk when clients are taking some psychotropic medications.

In some parts of the country, it can be hot any day of the year, and you are likely to be aware of how some medications lower the body's ability to reduce its core temperature. Prescribers in parts of the country with longer winters may need to remind clients to stay out of the heat to avoid heat exhaustion or heat stroke. Consider how to systematically warn all your clients on these medications when the seasons change.

Ginger ale may help a client who is nauseated from taking medication.

I tell clients complaining of nausea that they should try ginger ale. It has no side effects, and some find it helpful. Whether they are motivated to try tells me how bad their nausea is.

Sometimes, when it does not work, I use standard medications for nausea.

Carpal tunnel may be related to low thyroid function.

I have seen clients who complained of carpal tunnel symptoms, then said the condition resolved when their hypothyroidism was treated. Low thyroid causes multiple physical changes that combine to compress the median nerve as it goes through the tunnel.

Bruxism may be a clue that your client has ADHD.

There is an odd connection between bruxism and ADHD. If you have a client with bruxism, inquire about the symptoms of attention deficit hyperactivity disorder. Sometimes, the hyperactive motor activity manifests as teeth-grinding movement at night. Make sure they wear a night guard. There are many more people with bruxism who don't have ADHD.

Medications used for one disease have accidentally been found helpful for others.

Encourage your clients to get vaccinated for shingles. The pain and itch associated with shingles can be debilitating. Fortunately, there are some newer and more effective medications for it. I had an elderly client with shingles on the scalp who found topical doxepin helpful, even though doxepin is ordinarily used as an antidepressant and sleep aid.

A change in your client's attitude toward therapy may be related to a change in their finances.

Recognize the connection between a change in your client's behavior and a change in their financial state. It is wise to have a financial screening process in place to avoid starting with a client, only to find out that they can't afford your treatment. If that happens, continuity of care may require helping them find an affordable provider. Sometimes, a client's financial situation deteriorates during the treatment. When that happens, you may need to work out a payment schedule or see them until they can find treatment elsewhere.

Be transparent with clients about what is expected of them. For example, some therapists in private practice require a credit card before an appointment can be scheduled. Others require a credit card, indicating that if a client misses an appointment, there will be a charge for the missed appointment.

If you do not have a monopoly in your area, get an idea of whether other providers are participating in insurance programs. If you are in a small town with several large employers, know what insurance most employees have. Some electronic medical record software includes coding and billing applications.

I have found that billing services do not consider the payoff worth going after secondary insurance. Remember that if you accept insurance, it will take a while to be paid. It could be months before you see the income if you are starting. It would be best to consider the labor cost of processing the paperwork.

I would rather write off bad debt than risk irritating clients into filing malpractice suits because they feel abandoned or don't want to pay. I tell myself that I am enjoying the luxury of giving good care regardless of the client's ability to pay. I gradually became more careful about whom I accepted for treatment. If their life was unmanageable, I figured their finances were too.

Clients may want to be seen less often than you feel is clinically indicated. I suggest working with them to accept a lower rate rather than stretching the time between appointments and risking delivering substandard care.

A direct discussion that results in a payment plan the client can keep up with will prevent them from developing resentment and you from creating a large accounts receivable.

There are laws preventing providers from offering a different rate to the client than they bill the insurance company. After charging the same full rate and making legitimate efforts to collect, you may be allowed to write off the debt as bad. You will want to know what is permissible in your area.

As you become known for having expertise working with difficult clients, more complicated clients will be referred to you. Set limits on your referral sources when you have too many of a specific type of client. In that way, you can lessen the likelihood of developing burnout. It may take time to learn which clients are the best matches. Don't be too proud to refer out. Sometimes, your setup is not equipped to handle clients who need more intense treatment. Some clients need a team of treaters or inpatient treatment to ensure effective treatment.

In this chapter: I talk about some situations that are not predictable and can surprise you. Heat exhaustion from prolonged heat exposure while on antipsychotics is predictable enough that you should anticipate it and take preventive measures for clients on antipsychotics.

In the next chapter: You'll see that clients can be surprising. But life can be even more surprising.

Part 6

REMAIN PRESENT WITH SUFFERING CLIENTS

This section approaches suffering from several angles. It illustrates how your client's suffering might affect you. I offer some personal experiences related to faith and suffering. Philosophical views on suffering and dissatisfaction are discussed. The section presents some practical ideas about being with clients who suffer and how to help those who experience egoic dissatisfaction. It concludes with encouragement to pursue your own spiritual quest.

Chapter 37
Personal Perspectives on Suffering and Faith

This chapter draws on my subjective personal experiences to inspire you as you sit with your suffering clients.

Hearing about others' suffering affects you.

As a therapist, you will come to know and care about your clients. Hearing about their suffering and the suffering of those they love may leave you feeling sad. The injustice and trauma they experienced may anger you.

Sometimes, you don't realize just how much hearing about others' suffering affects you.

I once worked at a community mental health center with people who were getting progressively poorer and sicker as the economy worsened. First, they would come late because their car had broken down. Then, they would not have the gas for the car trip. Next, someone else would bring them because they had to sell their car. It would cause them to be late in getting their medications refilled.

Eventually, medication was less affordable because they had lost the job they couldn't get to. We would shift to a cheaper medication with more side effects. Later, they could not afford that, so we would use samples when available. But it was often not the best medication. After missed doses, missed appointments, and increasing financial stress, they would relapse into despair. All of this happened because of a lack of money and opportunity in a system underfunded by a public that did not care enough.

At about the same time, I went to a performance of *La Bohème* that dealt with the suffering of the poor. In the middle of an aria, I was suddenly overcome with uncontrollable sobbing for minutes. I had released all that pent-up sadness.

Sitting with clients in their suffering and experiencing it vicariously keeps me looking for an answer to why we suffer. I'm still looking. I want to share some experiences that have added to my understanding. I hope these experiences will help you as you work with suffering clients. Sometimes, after hearing so many accounts of suffering, you may feel like your soul hurts by the time you arrive home.

Now, I am taking off my therapist's hat.

If a client knows very little about you, what they project onto you in the transference is more reflective of them. Judiciously revealing things about yourself may sometimes be helpful in supportive therapy. But in more analytically oriented therapy, it would be more detrimental to introduce these artifacts into the transference. My sharing my story with you should not be taken as a suggestion that you share similar information with your clients.

When we see clients, they are often dispirited. Illness has physical, mental, and spiritual aspects. The spiritual aspect of clients' suffering is too essential for me to ignore, despite the topic's controversial and subjective nature.

You may not share many of my beliefs. That is okay. I hope, however, that you will not discount what I have written so far because of what you are about to read. I hope you will consider each point separately on its own merits. Please imagine this chapter as a way to open yourself to wonder.

As you read this chapter, remember what my Davidson College philosophy professor, Dr. George Abernathy, once told our class: "The surest road to irrelevance is a too great insistence on relevance."

Now, I am going to take off my therapist hat and speak to you person to person. I am moving from a deliberately factual, objective, scientific mode into a subjective one.

I am like one of the five blind men who each had a part of the elephant to describe but could not picture the whole elephant. I am going to tell you what part I have discovered. I am a work in progress, and my understanding is also a work in progress.

Skyline Drive was a turning point in my life.

Despite being raised by faithful Protestant parents who lived their beliefs, there have been times in my life when I would have described myself as an agnostic humanist who believed only in the scientific method.

A turning point came when I was on Skyline Drive in the Smoky Mountains. Looking over a valley at dusk, I told my girlfriend that I could imagine God looking down on the valley like the Jolly Green Giant. She told me I was fooling myself by thinking that I was an agnostic because I did not have it in me. She said that believing in God was part of the person I was, and I couldn't escape it. That was the beginning of my path back to believing.

I wish you could have
been at Conyers with me.

To avoid an argument, on October 13, 1998, I went with a family member to the grounds of Nancy Fowler's house in Conyers, Georgia, where a crowd had gathered. My family member had told me that Ms. Fowler was a nurse whom the Virgin Mary visited.

My family member told me that in the last apparition, the Virgin Mary told Nancy Fowler that this October visit would be the last time she would visit her. Hearing this, I said, "How clever of Ms. Fowler to get out of having hundreds of people trampling down her grass every month by saying that the Virgin Mary, and not she, was stopping this." I complained that I was missing a day's pay by having to go. Still, I knew that if I did not go, I would never hear the end of it.

So I went. I was there at noon with crowds of people who were sitting on lawn chairs surrounding Nancy Fowler's house. Some were using their Polaroid cameras to take pictures of the sun. They showed the photos to each other and commented on the stairway in the image. I thought it was an artifact of the camera's aperture and that they were fooling themselves.

I looked at the sun. It was the same sun I'd seen before. It was too bright to look at, and it was the same size as always. Nothing new. I noticed the sky was a clear Carolina blue with no clouds in sight. It was just about noon.

I had my back to the sun when I heard a roar from the crowd. I turned around to find that the sun had shrunk to about one-tenth its size and that I could look at it without hurting my eyes. It spun in place, and clouds gradually emerged simultaneously from the right and left sides. I asked myself what I was looking at. It did not look like an eclipse. I asked myself if the sun was really that small. Yes, it was. I questioned if it was really turning. Yes, it was. Were the clouds really emerging on either side? Yes.

It lasted about ten minutes. It was long enough for me to stop myself several times and recheck my observations. I also asked myself if I was in an altered state and decided I was not. Then the sun returned to looking like its regular self, and I could not look at it directly. The clouds were still there.

My family member used her Canon camera to take several pictures of it. When the film was developed, the sun was shrunken, just as I had seen it, and the sun took up a very small space on the film. I still have one of the photos. You will see the photo on my website: jeffduffeymdbooks.com

At about the same time at which the sun reverted to its ordinary shape, an announcement came over the loudspeaker attached to Nancy Fowler's house. The announcer said the Virgin Mary had just appeared to Nancy Fowler in the room set aside for that purpose.

A person took notes of what was said. Nancy Fowler had noticed that the Virgin Mary had tears coming down her face. Nancy Fowler asked her why she was crying. The Virgin Mary said that our suffering moved her and God, and that they were with us in our suffering. She said things would get worse before they got better, but to hang on because they would get better. The Virgin Mary told Nancy Fowler that she and God were pleased that people had come.

I don't remember all that was relayed on the loudspeaker. I could hardly believe what had just happened. I realized I had always had doubts about God and Jesus because it just seemed too good to be true. I grew up in church and studied religion in college, but it felt abstract. Now I had seen the sun shrink before my very eyes, and the message of the Virgin Mary dovetailed with what I had been taught.

God was real. How wonderful! I felt like a baby relinquishing some of its omnipotence, having realized it has a loving parent. I realized that I would no longer get to make up my own rules and decided to reexamine the Bible in the light of my experience.

I believe God does not intend for us to suffer. God is with us in our suffering. God gives us free will, and we make mistakes and live in a world so complex that bad things sometimes accidentally happen. We need to accept that suffering is part of life. Some of our suffering is man-made, and that is the part that may be amenable to therapy.

Science is also a belief system.

I eventually came to realize that scientists also have a belief system. They believe something is not valid unless it can be proven scientifically. They agree that science is the only way of knowing. They are disciples of science.

We owe so much to science, but its domain is the natural. After my experience at Conyers, I realized there is a supernatural that is beyond science.

Suspension bridges are mysterious to me, but I don't have to understand them to cross.

I have mentioned my dog, Sophie, and you may have seen her in my YouTube videos about college: https://www.youtube.-com/playlist?list=PL8Hb1mIKF05i5KhUX_8zAs4LD783Rd3sH Or google "YouTube How to Get Ready for College in Trying Times Duffey."

Sophie's experience walking in the neighborhood with me differs significantly from mine. She smells so many things that I cannot smell and hears noises I cannot hear. On the other hand, I see colors she cannot appreciate. So her reality differs from mine. This difference makes me think there is more than meets the eye. It suggests that there is more than one way of experiencing reality.

I am reminded of what an Episcopal priest said when asked about transubstantiation. He said Catholics believe that when the priest blesses the bread and wine, they are transformed into the body and blood of Christ. He said Methodists believe the bread and wine symbolize Christ's body and blood. When asked what Episcopalians believe, he said they believe it is a mystery, which is okay.

I have become comfortable with many things being mysterious and still being okay. There are also things I don't understand, and that is okay. For example, I don't understand the physics of suspension bridges, but I cross them anyway.

My parents showed me
what God's love is like.

I feel like we might not be capable of comprehending God, but we can experience God. God is ineffable. God, humanity, and life defy reductionist theories. This book is an example of those limitations.

I think I experienced what God is like by having such wonderful parents. They were stricter on me when I was a little kid and did not know better. As I matured, they gave me more freedom, and I did the right thing not out of fear of punishment, but out of love for my parents and the recognition that they loved me and had sacrificed for me.

Growing up, I did not always understand why my parents did certain things, but I came to realize that they had my interests at heart. They knew they could not control or prearrange my path, so they provided me with opportunities to gain experience and tried to teach and prepare me for the path.

Looking back on my adolescence, I realize my parents lost sleep worrying about me as I dated, but they allowed me to learn from my mistakes. They wanted me to be myself, and their love and acceptance, graciously given, were empowering. I did not fully appreciate their wisdom or sacrifices until I was older. I have found that clients whose parents were not like mine have a more challenging time believing in a loving God.

I believe Father James Finley described the nature of God's love best in the passage quoted earlier. To repeat, he said, "We are most powerless in being powerless to be anything else other than infinitely loved by God" (Moon 2016).

The gestalt of faith helps you not overlook other clues that suggest there is more than meets the eye.

Have you ever driven into a public park and seen a sign that asked you to tune your radio to a subcarrier radio frequency to listen to directions? If you tune in, you might hear a faint voice giving you information about the park through all the static of the stronger radio stations. I like to think that God's spirit is like that subcarrier station. It is always there in the background if we can tune out all the world's distractions. Hearing it is the benefit of having an attentive mindset.

Sometimes, clues that there is more than meets the eye arise when things that seem beyond serendipity happen. Time after time, one client would tell me something improbable, like they had solved their problem of their ears turning green by eating carrots cooked with sauerkraut. Then, the next client would complain that their ears were turning green. The first client had presented me with the unlikely solution to the second client's problem.

For another example, I had a client come in and complain that the Paxil they were taking made it take too long to have an orgasm. Later that day, a client came in and complained about premature ejaculation. I told them to switch the antidepressant to Paxil.

Another client told me their antidepressant seemed to reduce their sensitivity to touch and interfered with the effectiveness of foreplay. That afternoon, yet another client complained about the sensation of something crawling underneath their skin. So I switched them to the first client's medication, which helped. The second client's formication-like symptom responded quickly, raising questions in my mind and making me think the underlying dynamics might be unusual.

Not infrequently, I see a client who has an unusual symptom complex I would not have ordinarily known about, except that I had read an obscure article about it the night before. When I pursued the workup, I found I was correct, and the article helped me know what to do.

You may experience a sense of transcendence when listening to music, viewing art, meditating, experiencing the wondrous complexity of nature, making love, or reading poetry. These activities may help your client who is suffering.

In some AA meetings, the compassion and grace are so palpable that the meeting seems like a manifestation of the sacred. Recovering alcoholics find redemption and healing through AA. AA members don't just recognize that the organization exists; they have faith that having it be part of their life can help them in their daily struggle to maintain sobriety.

People may struggle to make the leap of faith from believing in God to believing that God can be an active part of their lives. Paul Tillich has written about this in his book *Courage to Be*.

Lean out over the hill.

An experience skiing showed me the benefit of faith.

Once, I was an awkward klutz who hated to fall and feared heights. I was dating an attractive woman who loved to ski. I had to take lessons if I was going to ski alongside her.

When people first learn how to ski, they learn to do the snow plow by positioning their skis like a V in front of them. This positioning feels natural as they are pushing against the gravity that would make them go down the hill faster.

In my first lesson on how to ski parallel, the instructor discussed using the edges of our skis to control our direction and velocity. He explained the principles of weighting and unweighting. He told me to lean out over my skis toward downhill. That would place my weight forward down the hill. That was the last thing I wanted to do. I knew I would go too fast, lose control, and fall down this steep hill in front of me.

But with my instructor's encouragement, I started to do it. The first sense of not being in control fueled my doubt, and I quickly leaned back and felt off balance. My instructor gently reassured me by explaining the paradox that I would be in more control if I leaned forward. I tried again and was surprised to find that I could control the skis even better than the snow plow and that my edges suddenly worked for me.

Not only did it all fit together, but it was a totally different skiing experience than using the snow plow. If I had not had faith in my ski instructor, I would never have tried it. Nor would I have known the pleasure of parallel skiing. I am proud to say I skied in the Alps some years later.

Another clue to there being more than meets the eye happens when, over the years, you repeatedly find that clients who were not expected to improve get well.

In this chapter: I discussed my personal perspective on suffering and faith.

In the next chapter: I will talk about how suffering raises existential issues.

Chapter 38
Philosophical Perspectives on Suffering

It is helpful to look at your client's suffering from different perspectives.

Suffering raises existential issues.

When I think of suffering, I think of uncontrollable situations, like the loss of a loved one, natural disasters, chronic pain, or catastrophic illness. The client and the therapist cannot alter the situation. Suffering makes people feel powerless and may raise existential questions.

Discovering your client's religious beliefs can help you call on these beliefs to provide a context for understanding their suffering and help them see the bigger picture.

Some clients view suffering as punishment they had coming. Therapy may help them not take suffering personally, but see it as a universal life experience, like aging.

For example, Buddhists might say, "There is suffering," rather than "I suffer." Buddhists believe we can know of suffering without objectifying it.

Elizabeth Mattis-Namgyel, in her book *The Power of an Open Question: The Buddha's Path to Freedom*, writes, "The shape of our life has less to do with what we encounter than with our relationship to it. When we objectify experience—be it beauty or pain—we enter into a relationship of struggle with our world—a world all about 'me.'"

She also writes, "The transformative aspect of suffering comes about through the realization that we're big enough to face this inevitable aspect of life."

Sitting with your client in their suffering shows them they don't have to avoid it and are not facing it alone. Your presence with them in the felt experience of their suffering shows them that the feeling is possibly bearable.

You may feel frustrated that there is nothing concrete you can do. Don't underestimate the power of just being with your client. Just being there is a behavioral statement about your ability to be with their suffering. As you help them identify and express their feelings, you show that you are comfortable hearing them. You may be the only one currently able to listen to them.

I am reminded of an experiment where patients undergoing surgery had volunteers hold their hands throughout the operation. The research showed that the patients whose hands were held had more positive post-operative courses than those whose hands were not held.

As you help your clients who may be going through stages of grief, you demonstrate your willingness to stay present. Remember that your clients will be susceptible to anything in your personal life that might suggest you won't be able to be there for them. Planned vacations and appointments you have canceled because of illness, surgeries, or accidents can trigger issues of abandonment in grieving clients.

If you review your client's history, you may identify other tragedies they have gotten through. Asking them how they did it reminds them of their strengths and resilience. Did they go through a time when they thought nothing would change, but after a time, it did? Who helped them get through those tragedies? Who can they reconnect with to help them now?

I understand that when a Jewish person dies, it is customary for the family to sit shiva for several days as people come to pay their respects. Being together for an extended time can be a transformative experience for family members, helping them navigate their shared grief.

As you listen to your clients describe their situation, look for other things going right in their lives. In that way, they realize that their suffering does not permeate every aspect of life. Is there something they are looking forward to doing? Would it be helpful to plan a future activity to look forward to?

It may seem trite to suggest entertainment, but a client experiencing almost unbearable suffering will welcome any distraction you might suggest. Movies, sports events, and television programs that capture their attention can take their mind off the situation and pass the time. You will find a list of funny movies in the book *Help Me Live:20 Things People with Cancer Want You to Know* by Lori Hope.

The egoic self is a source of dissatisfaction.

I have a meditation cushion in my home office. But, unfortunately, my dog spends more time on it than I do. Neither of us has reached enlightenment, and I think Sophie may be in the lead. All kidding aside, I want to share my limited understanding of Buddhist concepts, which might help you work with clients.

Reading about Buddhism without practicing meditation is like a virgin reading about sex and thinking they understand it. I can't speak to direct experience because I have not meditated enough to have had direct experience. Still, I suspect that understanding may come more from the modality of direct experience rather than the modality of conventional knowing/thinking.

I find parallels between Buddhist meditation and centering, contemplative prayer. In *The Wisdom Jesus: Transforming Heart and Mind—A New Perspective on Christ and His Message*, Cynthia Bourgeault refers to "a pathway of perception 'epinoia'—knowing through intuition and direct revelation, not through linear didactic logic" (Bourgeault 2008).

While my Conyers experience brought home the reality of God, I have found Buddhist concepts helpful in understanding how self-centered, egoistic thinking leads to dissatisfaction. I think therapists and Buddhists share a common wish: People should be able to put aside their self-centeredness to have a more direct experience of life and interconnectedness.

Centuries before Freud, Buddhists asked questions about the nature of suffering. English translators have taken the word for *dissatisfaction* and translated it into the English word *suffering*. The egoic self is seen as the source of dissatisfaction. When Buddhists renounce the egoic self, they let go of holding back.

This state of egolessness is roughly somewhat parallel to the Christians who, confident in being accepted and loved by God, no longer worry about themselves. They are then freed up to love and connect with those around them while experiencing what Cynthia Bourgeault describes as "God's aliveness."

Buddhists take egolessness a step further and apply it to the universe.

Children are separate from their fathers, but, as children, they share likeness and closeness. Christians believe they are children of God. So they believe there are two entities—God and the children of God. That makes other people brothers and sisters, also made in the image of God.

Buddhists believe in the non-duality of the universe. They believe that when you peel off the ego, what is underneath is part of one sacred basic goodness and that the solidity of a separate self is an illusion. Buddhists rest in this basic goodness, this cradle of loving kindness, which allows them to be content in the face of the fearfulness of life's uncertainty, vastness, and impermanence. They can know things without objectifying them. Rather than having to be something apart, they are said to connect with a radiant wisdom and compassion at life's core. Being able to draw from basic goodness helps them avoid compassion fatigue.

In her book *The Power of the Open Question*, Elizabeth Mattis Namgyel writes, "Faith is the mind of an open question. And when we ask an open question, we don't get some kind of static answer. We don't arrive at a final destination or reach a definite conclusion we can hold to and say, 'That's it!' Faith is an experience, a way of being in life, that comes from a mind that does not reach conclusions about the world of things. So to stay with this bigger way of being without turning away is what it means to walk by faith" (Mattis-Namgyel 2011).

Christians rest in their experience of God's steadfast love.

While having different views of the sacred, the beliefs of both religious traditions value loving kindness, open-heartedness, and connectedness.

You can use the acronym *DisBlaLoPa* to remind you about what worries the egoistic self.

I have found the Buddhist concept of the eight worldly dharmas helpful in understanding what the egoistic self worries about. They are four sets of opposites. The egoistic self fears **dis**grace and hopes for admiration. It fears **bla**me and hopes for praise. It fears **lo**ss and hopes for gain. It fears **pa**in and hopes for pleasure.

Do you remember Ricky Martin's song "Livin' la Vida Loca"? *Vida loca* translates loosely as "crazy life." I like to say that our egos worry about the DisBlaLoPa.

As an exercise, try labeling your own thoughts for a couple of hours to see how many fall into one of these eight categories. The client doing such an exercise may realize how futile and unsatisfying this egoistic thinking is and what a dead-end experience the self-centered life is that clings to the ego.

If you become more adept at labeling *your* egoistic thoughts, you will be more alert when your clients express them. Through meditation, you may learn how to focus on your breath and how to relinquish unskillful thoughts and put skillful ones in their place, which may lead to peaceful contentment.

Seek, and ye shall find (Matthew 7:7).

The barn on my farm was filled with pigeons, which pooped all over the hay I fed to my sheep. Nothing I did seemed to get rid of the pigeons. I made the tough decision to shoot them. I lost a live bullet in my hay-filled barn. My four-year-old daughter was in that barn every day. So I needed to find a needle in a haystack. I spent hours examining the hay little by little for this tiny .22 caliber bullet. As I got closer and closer to having examined all the hay, I felt increasingly upset. Had I missed it?

Then, in the final clump of hay, I found the bullet. Simultaneously, I had a strong, almost overpowering, sense of knowing "Seek and ye shall find." It felt like I was being given a message to not give up on seeking in my life.

I hope that you, too, will continue your own spiritual quest. Having asked yourself the crucial questions, you will be better prepared to help your clients when they struggle with existential crises and you sit with them in their suffering.

These books may clarify and expand on some ideas introduced in this chapter.

- *A Call to Compassion: Bringing Buddhist Practices of the Heart into the Soul of Psychology* by Aura Glaser
- *Awakening Loving Kindness* by Pema Chodron
- *Beyond Happiness: The Zen Way to True Contentment* by Ezra Bayda
- *Christian Meditation: Experiencing the Presence of God* by James Finley
- *Don't Bite the Hook: Finding Freedom from Anger, Resentment, and Other Destructive Emotions* by Pema Chodron
- *Reiki A Torch in Daylight: A Guide for Spiritual Reiki* by Karyn K. Mitchell, ND, PhD
- *Shambhala: The Sacred Path of the Warrior* by Chogyam Trungpa
- *Start Where You Are: A Guide to Compassionate Living* by Pema Chodron
- *The Great Eastern Sun: The Wisdom of Shambhala* by Chogyam Trungpa
- *The Places That Scare You: A Guide to Fearlessness in Difficult Times* by Pema Chodron
- *The Power of an Open Question: The Buddha's Path to Freedom* by Elizabeth Mattis Namgyel
- *The Wisdom Jesus: Transforming Heart and Mind—A New Perspective on Christ and His Message* by Cynthia Bourgeault
- *Turning the Mind Into an Ally* by Sakyong Mipham
- *What Makes You Not a Buddhist* by Dzongsar Jamyang Khyentse

- *When Things Fall Apart: Heart Advice for Difficult Times* by Pema Chodron

---

In this chapter: I offered some ideas and experiences to help you with suffering clients.

In the next chapter: I will summarize the steps in understanding the client who baffles you.

Chapter 39
Summary

To understand your baffling client, you have explored the ins and outs of the therapeutic relationship, the key to psychotherapy.

This book has offered steps to understand your baffling client:

1. Find hidden patterns by taking an extensive history.
2. Identify the nature of your therapeutic relationship with your client.
3. Integrate the clues about your client from reflecting on:

A. The ways the client affects you
B. The emerging transference-countertransference
C. The events occurring in therapy
D. Their upbringing
E. Their dynamics
F. Their character type
G. Their life situations

4. Employ the therapeutic methods you have determined that best fit your client.
5. Negotiate the medical minefield, relying on accepted principles and the effective practice patterns you have established.
6. Abide with your profoundly suffering client even when there is nothing you can do to alleviate the outcome.

Many things have changed over the fifty years I have been working with clients. You will see even more changes, and they will occur faster. Yet your relationship with your client will always be essential in understanding your baffling client.

I appreciate your willingness to read this book and hope you will use it as a reference as opportunities arise.

Most authors can get an inkling of how their ideas were received by looking at the sales of their books. The multiple ways this book will be distributed mean that sales will not reflect your response. Would you let me know about your experience with this book? My email address is jeffduffeymd@gmail.com. I would appreciate it very much. Thanks.

Bibliography

The author does not endorse the content of the books or articles named in this book. The author does not provide any sort of guarantee that they are accurate, timely, or complete. The bibliography below does not repeat works listed in Chapter 19, Chapter 32, or those mentioned in the References.

Build the Life You Want: The Art and Science of Getting Happier by Arthur C. Brooks and Oprah Winfrey

Children of the Self-Absorbed: A Grown-Up's Guide to Getting Over Narcissistic Parents by Nina W. Brown

Choosing to Live: How to Defeat Suicide Through Cognitive Therapy by Thomas Ellis and Cory Newman

Clinical Manual for the Assessment and Treatment of Suicidal Patients by John Chiles, Kirk Strosahl, and Laura Weiss Roberts

Experiences in Groups and Other Papers by Wilfred R. Bion

Exploring Your Unplanned Pregnancy: Single Motherhood, Adoption, and Abortion Questions and Resources by Jeff Duffey

Hello to All That: A Memoir of War, Zoloft, and Peace by John Falk

Help Me Live, revised:20 Things People with Cancer Want You to Know by Lori Hope

Learning to Fly: Trapeze—Reflections on Fear, Trust, and the Joy of Letting Go by Sam Keen

Never Be Lied to Again by David J. Lieberman

Pathfinders: Overcoming the Crises of Adult Life and Finding Your Own Path to Well-Being by Gail Sheehy

People of the Lie: The Hope for Healing Human Evil by M. Scott Peck

Reclaiming Your Life After Rape: Cognitive-Behavioral Therapy for Posttraumatic Stress Disorder Client Workbook (Treatments That Work) by Barbara Olasov Rothbaum

Reviving Ophelia: Saving the Selves of Adolescent Girls by Mary Pipher and Ruth Ross

The Plant Paradox: The Hidden Dangers in "Healthy" Foods that Cause Disease and Weight Gain by Steven R. Gundry

Acknowledgments

Writing starts as a sometimes lonely, solitary pursuit that evolves into a collective effort as the work progresses. The coffee coaster on my desk reads, "The Worst Enemy to Creativity is Self-Doubt." I am deeply grateful to my family, friends, colleagues, and writers' group, who helped me overcome my self-doubt and improve my writing.

I am thankful for my wife, Barbara Roquemore, my North Star, whose patience and support never faltered. The insights Christy Roquemore, my stepdaughter, shared were invaluable.

At the Georgia College and State University Counseling Center, I worked with licensed professional counselors, advanced practice psychiatric nurses, social workers, marriage and family therapists, and a psychologist. I was fortunate to have representatives from my target audience who were willing to diligently read and critique my drafts and provide guidance. They include Shadisha Bennett-Brodie, Jenny Brooks, Karon Ferguson, Jamie Gray, Katherine Holtzclaw, Pam Jones, Jan Nodine, Evelyn Palm, Andrea Paugh, and Steve Wilson, PhD. They put in many hours to not only help me but also because they believed in the importance of therapy.

When writers begin a work, they worry that something will get in the way of completing it. It was great comfort to know that Susan Spencer, another GCSU Counseling Center colleague, was willing to take up the torch in my stead if need be. Her clinical wisdom and editorial skills are much appreciated.

My colleagues from other times also stepped up to help me: Lee Edwards, PhD, Barry Jones, MD, Laura Pilafas, and John McMillon.

I was thrilled to have readers representing the general public read my drafts. Included in these were Wendy Mourad, Keith Muse, and Barbara Buchwald.

I am indebted to *The Up and Cumming Writers Group*— Katrina Bak, Pam Barnard, Dylan Brons, Isa Caraballo, Jon Copsey, Katherine Eitel, Doug Horton, B. R. Marcus, Glenn Schendel, Brianna Schantz, Ashley Shaw, and Susan Starnes— for their meticulous, sentence-by-sentence, monthly critiques of my drafts. The moral support and the expertise they shared will not be forgotten.

It was a blessing to be able to rely on the wise advice and expertise of my editor, Kristy Phillips, who helped me with the final steps of bringing this book to life.

At times, I wanted to give up. Then I remembered that my supervisors at The Sheppard and Enoch Pratt Hospital had offered their timeless wisdom to me. It was my responsibility to pass it on to others who may not have been so incredibly lucky as to have had such experiences. I hope you will also pass on this information by sharing this book with others.

About the Author

I received a BS from Davidson College and an MD from the Medical College of Georgia. I did my psychiatric residency at Sheppard Pratt Hospital.

It cannot be emphasized enough what a gift it was to be trained by experienced psychotherapists, psychiatrists, and psychoanalysts at Sheppard Pratt Hospital outside Baltimore. Working there with inpatients in supervised treatment for several months at a time was a rare opportunity to get to know people deeply. I had other opportunities to do long-term treatment in various settings, including a residential treatment center for adolescents, a long-term rehab hospital for dual-diagnosed adolescents, intensive outpatient programs, and private practice. Training programs encourage residents to have therapy themselves. I've had a personal analysis, so I have been on the patient side of long-term therapy.

My short-term therapy experience came from working in several settings: a forensic unit, a US Public Health Service hospital, a Veterans Administration hospital alcohol treatment unit, an acute adult unit of a state psychiatric hospital, and community mental health centers.

Emory University, Mercer University, and the University of Maryland gave me opportunities to work with psychiatric residents and medical students as an associate clinical professor.

I worked as a psychiatrist for the Georgia College and State University counseling center for seventeen years. While there, I wrote *Exploring Your Unplanned Pregnancy* and co-authored *Search: A Guide for College and Life* with my wife, Dr. Barbara Roquemore, EdD.

Customer reviews make an incredible difference in how visible this book will be on Amazon and whether other therapists think it is worth buying. You can help other therapists find this book more readily by posting a review on Amazon. A sentence or two would be very much appreciated. Thank you.

Scan the QR code to leave a review.

Can you think of a colleague you could share your copy with?

References

American Foundation for Suicide Prevention (2018*)* "Is it possible to assess short-term risk of suicide?" https://afsp.org/story/is-it-possible-to-assess-short-term-risk-of-suicide/

Bailey R.& Pico J. (2023) "Defense mechanisms." *StatPearls Publishing*, 2025 Jan https://www.ncbi.nlm.nih.gov/books/NBK559106/

Bandler, R. & Grinder J. (1979) *Frogs into princes: Neurolinguistic programming.* Real People's Press

Berger, M., & Gray, J. & Roth, B. (2018). "The expanded biology of serotonin." *Annual Review of Medicine.* 2009;60:355–366. doi: 10.1146/annurev.med.60.042307.110802

Bojanic L. et al. (2020). "Early post-discharge suicide in mental health patients: Findings from a national clinical survey." *Frontiers in Psychiatry* 11:502. https://doi.org/10.3389/fpsyt.2020.00502

Bouregeault, C. (2008) *The wisdom Jesus: Transforming heart and mind- A new perspective on Christ and his message.* Shambhala Publications

Brown, N. (2020) *Children of the self-absorbed: A grownup's guide to getting over narcissistic parents.* New Harbinger Press

Chodron, P. (2022) *Don't bite the hook: Finding freedom from anger, resentment, and other destructive emotions.* Shambhala Publications

Cuncic, A. (2024) "Is Imposter Syndrome Holding You Back from Living Your Best Life?" *Verywellmind* https://www.verywellmind.com/imposter-syndrome-and-social-anxiety-disorder-4156469

Folstein, M., Folstein, S., & McHugh, P, (1975). "Mini-mental state: A practical method for grading the cognitive state of patients for the clinician." *Journal of Psychiatric Research*, 12(3),189-198 https://meded.temertymedicine.utoronto.ca/sites/default/files/assets/resource/document/mini-mental-state-examinationmmse.pdf

Forward, S. & Frazier, D. (2019) *Emotional blackmail: When the people in your life use fear, obligation, and guilt to manipulate you.* Harper Paperbacks

Friedman, S. (2006) "Shaping new behaviors" *Good Bird ™ Magazine,* Vol 2-1, 2006:16-18 www.goodbirdinc.com reprinted on the internet through Behavior Works https://www.behaviorworks.org/files/articles/Shaping%20New%20Behaviors.pdf

Furman, D. et al. (2019). "Chronic inflammation in the etiology of disease across the lifespan." *Nature Medicine,* Dec 5;*25,(12)*:1822-1832. doi: 10.1038/s41591-019-0675-0

Gill, J.D. (2022) *Doing psychotherapy: A primer.* Kindle Direct Publishing

Greenson, R (1959) The classic psychoanalytic approach. In S. Arieti (ed.)

Hertz, R. (2012) T*hat's Disgusting: Unraveling the Mysteries of Repulsion.* W.W. Norton & Company

Hooley, J., Fox et al (2020) "Nonsuicidal self-injury: Diagnostic challenges and current perspectives." *Neuropsychiatric Disease and Treatment.* 2020 Jan 10;16:101–112. doi: 10.2147/NDT.S198806

Hope, L, (2011) *Help me live: 20 things people with cancer want you to know.* Clarkson Potter/Ten Speed.

Huecker, M. et al. (2023) "Imposter Phenomenon" *National Library of Medicine Stat Pearls* https://www.ncbi.nlm.nih.gov/books/NBK585058/

Kahn, J., & Veras, B. (2022, March) "Psychosis: The 5 Comorbidity-defined subtypes." *Current Psychiatry.* 2022 March;21(3):22-31 | doi: 10.12788/cp.0221

Kaplan, A. (2011, May 23) "Can a suicide scale predict the unpredictable?" *Psychiatric Times* https://www.psychiatrictimes.com/view/can-suicide-scale-predict-unpredictable

Kreisman, J., & Straus, H. (2021) *I hate you don't leave me: Understanding the borderline personality.* Third Edition. *Tarcher Perigree*

Main, T. (1957) "The ailment." *The British Journal of Medical Psychology* 30 (3) 129-145 https://bpspsychub.onlinelibrary.wiley.com/doi/abs/10.1111/j.2044-8341.1957.tb01193.x

Markova, D., (2021) *I will not die an unlived life: Reclaiming purpose and passion (find yourself and live life at the fullest).* Conari Press

Mason, P., & Kreger, R. (2020) *Stop walking on eggshells: Taking your life back when someone you care about has borderline personality disorder.* Third Edition. New Harbinger Publications

Mattis-Namgyel, E. (2011) *The power of an open question: The Buddha's path to freedom.* Shambhala Publications

Moon, G. (2006) "Christian Meditation: Experiencing the presence of God: An interview with James Finley." *The Martin Institute*

Myth@neurowonderful. "The five neurodivergent love languages" *Stimpunks Foundation* https://stimpunks.org/2022/01/22/the-five-neurodivergent-love-languages-2/.

Namie, G., & Namie, R. (2009) *The bully at work: what you can do to stop the hurt and reclaim your dignity on the job.* Sourcebooks

Nasreddine, Z. (2024) "Montreal Test of Cognitive Ability," *Moca Cognition* https://www.mocacognition.com/the-moca-test/

References

Neo, P. (2023) "How to break up with a narcissist:12 tips+What to expect." *Mindbodygreen* https://www.mindbodygreen.com/articles/breaking-up-with-a-narcissist

Nowinski, J. (1989) *A Lifelong Love Affair: Keeping Sexual Desire Alive in Your Relationship.* Olympic Marketing Corp

O'Bryan, A. (2022) "How to practice active listening:16 Examples and techniques." *Positive Communication* https://positivepsychology.com/active-listening-techniques/

Payne, R., (2018) *A framework for understanding poverty: A cognitive approach.* Aha! Press

Pier, K., & Marin, L. (2016) "The neurobiology of borderline personality disorder." *Psychiatric Times*, Mar 31:33,(3 .https://www.psychiatrictimes.com/view/neurobiology-borderline-personality-disorder

Reekum, R. et al. (2005) "Apathy: Why care?" *Psychiatryonline* https://psychiatryonline.org/doi/full/10.1176/jnp.17.1.7)

Roquemore, B. & Duffey, J. (2020) *Search: A guide to college and life.* Cairde, Karuna,& Hedd Publishing LLC

Rutherford, M. (2014) *The artisan teacher: A field guide to skillful teaching.* Lighting Source

Sarai S., Mekala H., Lippmann S. "Lithium suicide prevention: A brief review and reminder." (2018) *Innov Clin Neurosci.* 2018 Nov 1;15(11-12):30-32. PMID: 30834169; PMCID: PMC6380616

Schofield, W. (2018) *Psychotherapy: The purchase of friendship Routledge.* First published in 1964

Stadje, R. et al. (2016) "The differential diagnosis of tiredness: A systemic review." *BMC Family Practice* . doi: 10.1186/s12875-016-0545-5

Streeja , V. et.al (2024) "Pharmacogenetics of selective serotonin reuptake inhibitors (SSRI): A serotonin reuptake transporter (SERT) based approach." *Neurochemistry International,* Feb;(173) 10567 https://www.sciencedirect.com/science/article/abs/pii/S0197018623002000

The American Handbook of Psychiatry. pp 1399–1415. Basic Books

van der Hart, O. (2012) "The use of imagery in phase 1 treatment of clients with complex dissociative disorders." *European Journal of Psychotraumatology,* 3(1). https://doi.org/10.3402/ejpt.v3i0.8458 or https://pmc.ncbi.nlm.nih.gov/articles/PMC3402145/

Vaughan, D. (1990) *Uncoupling: Turning points in intimate relationships.* Knopf Doubleday Publishing Group

Weiss, R. (1975) *Marital Separation: Coping with the end of a marriage and the transition to being single.* Basic Books

References

Wendling, P. "Four biologically, clinically distinct autism subtypes." *Medscape* 2025 Jul 16

Yaseen, Z. et al. (2012) "Emergency room validation of the revised Suicide Trigger Scate (STS-3): a measure of a hypothesized suicide trigger state." *Pub Med* https://pubmed.ncbi.nlm.nih.gov/23024805/

Yehuda, R., & Lehrner A. (2018) "Intergenerational transmission of trauma effects: Putative role of epigenetic mechanisms." *World Psychiatry*, Oct;17(3)243-257 https://onlinelibrary.wiley.com/doi/10.1002/wps.20568

Zhu J, Klein-Fedyshin M, Stevenson J.M. "Serotonin Transporter Gene Polymorphisms and Selective Serotonin Reuptake Inhibitor Tolerability: Review of Pharmacogenetic Evidence." *Pharmacotherapy.* 2017 Sep;37(9):1089-1104. doi: 10.1002/phar.1978. Epub 2017 Aug 11. PMID: 28654193. https://pubmed.ncbi.nlm.nih.gov/28654193/

Appendix

This appendix first lists resources and educational materials for working with college students, and then for working with diverse people of all ages.

Resources for your diverse college student clients

The following website not only contains support resources but describes assistive technology available for students with autism, cognitive deficits, hearing deficits, ADHD, and other physical disabilities. https://www.affordablecollegesonline.org/college-resource-center/resources-for-students-with-disabilities/

American Muslim Health Professionals indicates that they are concerned with advocacy, health education, and career development. Moreover, they are an empowerment organization. They note they have an outreach of seven thousand health professionals and students working to leverage the educational background and skills of Muslims in the health care sector to improve the health of Americans.

The Asperger/Autism Network (AANE) indicates that they "work with individuals, families, and professionals to help people with Asperger Syndrome and similar autism spectrum profiles building meaningful, connected lives." Find more at https://www.aane.org

Campus Pride is a national nonprofit organization for student leaders and campus groups. It works to develop a safer college environment for LGBT students. https://www.campuspride.org

Gender Diversity provides education and support services and can use Skype for individual consultations. http://www.genderdiversity.org/individual-support/

The Center for Global Education: An international resource center lists programs available for international students.

The College Autism Network puts together people who are working to help college students on the autism spectrum have a better college experience and improve their access and success. Investigate at https://collegeautismnetwork.org

LGBT National Help Center, which also has a hotline (888-843-4564) and youth chat line serving youth through age twenty-five (800-246-7743). Their link is https://www.glbthotline.org/

Lost-n-Found Youth assists homeless LGBT youth and is based in Atlanta, Georgia

The National Society of Black Engineers is a sizeable student-run organization that seeks to provide personal and professional opportunities for success by improving the recruitment and retention of Black and other minority engineers. http://nsbe.org/

SACNAS indicates it is "an inclusive organization dedicating to fostering the success of Chicanos/Hispanics and Native Americans, from college students to professionals, in attaining advanced degrees, careers, and positions of leadership in STEM." Web source: https://www.sacnas.org/who-we-are/mission-impact/

Many colleges offer **SafeSpace training programs** to students and faculty who want to learn more about the transgender community, available resources, and how to be an ally best.

The Steve Fund is dedicated to the mental health and emotional well-being of students of color. You can text 741741 to talk to a live, trained crisis counselor. They have a Knowledge Center as well. Look up www.stevefund.org

Resources for students
and non-students alike:

Everything You Ever Wanted to Know About Trans* (But Were Afraid to Ask) by Brynn Tannehill is as comprehensive as its title suggests.

At **NAMI**'s website (https://www.nami.org/Find-Support/LGBTQ) you will find leads to multiple resources and a discussion of the stressors facing members of the LGBTQIA community. The site can help you if you want to locate an LGBTQIA-inclusive provider. The site mentions the Trevor Project. It has a toll-free twenty-four-hour national suicide hotline for LGBTQIA youth, which is 866-488-7386. The **Trevor Project** site is https://www.thetrevorproject.org/. They have online chat and confidential text messaging. To chat, you link to http://www.thetrevorproject.org/pages/get-help-now#tc or text "Trevor" to 202-304-1200 for confidential text messaging.

PFLAG's website notes that PFLAG offers support, education, and advocacy to unite LGBT people with family, friends, and allies and advance equality. https://pflag.org/
If you would like more knowledge about the LGBTQ community and help with being an ally for the community, check out Straight for Equality at http://www.straightforequality.org/about

Trans Lifeline is a national crisis hotline for transgender people in the United States staffed entirely by other trans and non-binary people. Their number is 877-565-8860.

Questionnaire Suggestions

You may want to choose among these commonly asked questions to create your own questionnaire for your initial evaluations. These questions are an accumulation from various sources I have read over the years and are not original with me.

Present Illness

Please describe what prompted you to come to see me. (For example, do you have symptoms that trouble you, worries, hurts, regrets, resentments, fears, or life questions?)

Past Psychiatric Treatment

If you have ever been an inpatient at a psychiatric hospital, please list places and dates.

If you have ever seen an outpatient counselor, psychologist, social worker, minister, or psychiatrist for any past nervous problems, please list them. Give dates as close as possible and describe why you saw them.

If you have ever had any psychological testing, please list dates and locations.

Medical History

- Are you allergic to any medication?
- Do you have other allergies (for example, hay fever, food allergies)?
- Please list all surgical operations you have had.
- Please list all medications you are currently taking. Include over-the-counter medications, herbs, and other health foods.
- Please list your physicians. When was your last physical examination?

If you have a history of a symptom, circle it:

- Have you ever been knocked out or lost consciousness (from a fall, playing sports, an accident, blow to the head)?
- Mononucleosis?
- Bad taste and burning sensation in your throat at night when you lie down that seems to come up from your stomach?
- Regular pains in your jaw joint; does it pop or click?
- Muscles that ache constantly?
- Do you have an infection or virus?
- Periods of diarrhea mixed with constipation?
- Asthma?
- Tired all the time?
- Do you have frequent headaches?
- Do you have migraine headaches?
- Diabetes?
- Sinus problems?

- High blood pressure?
- Heart attack?
- Irregular heartbeats?
- Other heart problems?
- Chest pain?
- Swelling in your legs or puffiness under your eyes?
- Cough?
- Tuberculosis?
- Short of breath?
- Glaucoma?
- Cancer?
- Inflammation of the liver (hepatitis)?
- Lupus?
- Arthritis?
- Pain at the top of your stomach after eating, like an ulcer?
- Recurrent urinary tract infection?
- Have you ever had a miscarriage or therapeutic abortion?
- How often do you menstruate in a year?
- Is there pain when you menstruate, and how much pain?
- Do you have any black hair on your abdomen, breasts, face, or back?
- Have you noticed your hair line is receding or that you are losing hair?

<u>Circle any of these symptoms that suggest decreased thyroid hormone:</u>

- Low body temperature
- Pulse below 60

- Hair changes
- Loss of eyebrows
- Puffy eyes
- Swollen legs
- Shortness of breath
- Low body temperature

Has anyone in your family died suddenly from irregular heartbeats or had a problem with irregular heartbeats?

Have you traveled outside the United States? Where? Are you exposed to well water, hazardous chemicals or fumes?

Do you have problems with your vision?

Do you have problems with your hearing?

When was the last time you felt suicidal? (This is intentionally a leading question.)

What role has violence played in your life?

Past Psychiatric Medication History

If you have ever taken any medication in the past from you family physician or from a psychiatrist for nervous problems or for depression, please list them, along with your response and any major side effects they gave you.

How often do you drink alcohol?

Have you had any problems from drinking?

When you drink alcohol, do you have trouble limiting how much you drink?

After drinking, do you ever have problems remembering what happened?

What role have illicit drugs, including marijuana, played in your life?

Developmental History

Where were you born?

Did your mother have trouble with labor or delivery?

Were you born prematurely?

From what you have heard people say, did you crawl, walk, and talk around the same age as other children?

If you were adopted, how old were you then?

If you were adopted, how old are your adoptive parents and what is your relationship like with them? Are your adoptive parents of the same sex?

Family History

How old is your biological mother, and how would you describe her and your relationship?

How old is your biological father, and how would you describe him and your relationship?

If you parents divorced, how old were you when it happened?

Did you have a stepmother, and what role did she play in your life?

Did you have a stepfather, and what role did he play in your life?

Please list your sisters, half-sisters, and stepsisters. Where do they live, and how are they doing? What are they like?

Please list your brothers, half-brothers, and stepbrothers. Where do they live, and how are they doing? What are the like?

How much were your grandparents involved in your life?

Do you have children? What are their ages?

Is there a history in your family of members being sad, depressed, anxious, or having problems with drugs or alcohol? If so, who?

Relationship History

What is your relationship status? Has there been a recent breakup? What can you say about your current and past relationships?

School History

What has school been like for you? What kind of grades did you make? Did you make friends easily? Did you play sports? Were you bullied?

Job History

What jobs have you had and what were they like? Were you harassed at work? How did you come to leave them?

What else do you need to tell me that has not been asked?

Review of Symptoms

Check the items that apply to how you have been recently:

- Feel irritable
- Feel sad or down
- Feel consistently more tired than I usually do
- Worry about my body and health more than usual for me.
- Don't enjoy things like I used to
- Don't eat nearly as much as I used to
- Eat for comfort more

- Are sleeping too much
- Are having trouble falling or staying asleep
- Feel worthless and am quicker to criticize myself
- Find myself feeling guilty a lot
- Read all of these first, then check the one or two answers that fit you the best:
- I have no suicidal thoughts.
- I feel like cutting or burning myself, but I don't have any interest in killing myself.
- Under a lot of pressure, I may briefly feel I would rather be dead than have to handle things sometimes.
- Suicidal thoughts go through my head but I don't feel like I really want to die.
- More and more, I am having intrusive suicidal thoughts that trouble me.
- I have unbearable feeling states, but I know they will pass and I can cope with them.
- I have unbearable feeling states and it seems like suicide is the only way to cope with them.
- I have spent some time recently thinking about how to kill myself.
- I intend to kill myself one day.
- I have decided on a plan to kill myself.
- I have thought about killing myself and started to act on my impulse but stopped.
- I have tried to kill myself recently but few if any people know it.
- I have made suicide attempts in the past.

Check this if you can access a firearm belonging to you or someone else ____

<u>Circle those that apply:</u>

- My sexual drive is less
- Friends are tired of asking me to go with them because I keep saying no
- I find myself crying often
- I seem to be spending a lot of time caught up in thinking depressive thoughts over and over

Have you had an episode when several of these four symptoms happened all at once? Check any that may apply:

- Difficulty breathing
- Dread
- Pounding heart
- Nervousness

<u>Circle the items that apply:</u>

- Feel nervous and anxious
- Feel tense
- Feel restless
- Feel like I have to be vigilant and on guard for some reason
- Space out for several minutes or more and can't remember what happened while I was feeling emotionally numb
- Am easily startled
- Certain things frighten me much more than other people
- Am in the habit of avoiding a lot of situations that others don't need to avoid

- Feel like something bad is going to happen
- Worry constantly
- Can't seem to control my worrying
- Find myself thinking about things over and over

<u>Circle these items if you know you are doing these too much but feel anxious if you don't do them:</u>

- Checking
- Washing
- Counting
- Cleaning
- Ordering
- Keeping things that should be thrown out
- Resisting temptations to do things that you know you don't really want to do

<u>Circle situations where you show at least moderate anxiety:</u>

- I am at least moderately anxious in social situations like eating in public, talking to teachers, going to a party, talking with people I don't know well, giving a report.
- I avoid groups.
- I don't raise my hand in class even when I am prepared.
- I fear being embarrassed.
- I am nervous in crowds
- I get nervous when I have to take a test or perform in some way.

<u>To what extent have emotional symptoms disrupted your (A) social, (B) family, or (C) school life?</u>

A. mildly, moderately, markedly, extremely
B. mildly, moderately, markedly, extremely
C. mildly, moderately, markedly, extremely

<u>Has there ever been a specific separate period of time (several days or week) when you were not your usual self and you had several of these symptoms at the same time: (Circle the items that apply)</u>

- You had much less sleep but lots more energy and were more busy and productive
- You were excessively happy to the point of being euphoric
- You talked very rapidly and seemed unable to stop talking
- You engaged in risky behavior even when not drinking
- You were in a very bad mood
- You overestimated your skills and what you could do or how important you are

If you want to explain something you have checked by describing it more, then write it here:

<u>This part of the questionnaire has to do with problems you may have with learning and attention. Circle items that apply.</u>

- When listening in class or at work, your mind repeatedly drifts off, or loses focus, missing cues or information you want to get

- Excessive difficulty getting started on tasks, e.g. homework, contacting people.
- Keep noticing your mind frequently drifts when you read
- Pastel backgrounds irritate you (trick question to catch over-endorsers)
- Often are easily distracted or sidetracked, disrupt a task in progress and switch to doing something else which is less important
- You have difficulty in comprehending and retaining things so you must read things many times over and over before you can commit them to memory or put the ideas together in your mind. You do this so much it takes you much more time to study.
- Forgetful in daily activities like turning off appliances, getting things at the store, returning phone calls, keeping appointments, paying bills, doing assignments
- Were born left handed and your parents made you change to use your right (trick question)
- So scattered you're late for friends, forget appointments, lose track of your money
- Seem more impulsive than other people
- Crawled later than other kids did
- Do not finish things
- Seem to always be moving or feel the need to move, tap, twist, wiggle
- Friends often ask you if you are listening to them
- Do not follow through with instructions
- Frequently avoid tasks that require a lot of mental effort
- Are always losing things

- Frequently are over-talkative
- May blurt out things before thinking
- Interrupt others who are talking
- Have difficulty waiting in lines
- Are a restless sleeper, kick your bedmate, or throw the covers off
- Grind your teeth
- Simply must study or work in a quiet setting because you are easily distracted otherwise
- Need to have noise in the background
- Nervous thoughts repeatedly interrupt you when you try to read
- Have family members who struggle with similar symptoms in school

Pick just one:

- Looking back at it now, you wonder if you may have had these symptoms all your life but are just noticing them now because school or work is harder
- You are sure you clearly had these symptoms as a child and others noticed them
- These symptoms became a problem first in middle or high school
- You first noticed these symptoms only after a time when you became depressed or anxious or were injured
- Haven't noticed these symptoms before now